NURSING'S RELATIONSHIP WITH MEDICINE

Do Siobhán agus Ewan.

Seo an sórt bualtraí a scríobh bhur n-athair.

Nursing's Relationship With Medicine

A Critical Realist Ethnography

SAM PORTER
Department of Sociology and Social Policy
Queen's University of Belfast

Avebury

Aldershot · Brookfield USA · Hong Kong · Singapore · Sydney

Published by
Avebury
Ashgate Publishing Ltd
Gower House
Croft Road
Aldershot
Hants GU11 3HR
England

Ashgate Publishing Company
Old Post Road
Brookfield
Vermont 05036
USA

British Library Cataloguing in Publication Data

Porter, Sam
    Nursing's Relationship with Medicine:
    Critical Realist Ethnography
    I. Title
    362.173   14, 519

ISBN 1 85972 209 1 ✓

Library of Congress Catalog Card Number: 95-80522

Printed and bound in Great Britain by Ipswich Book Co. Ltd., Ipswich, Suffolk

Contents

Acknowledgements

Though readers may find it hard to believe, the ideas set out in this book have been five years in the making. During that time, I have published drafts of my arguments in a number of journals. I would like to thank the editors and publishers of the following journals for giving me permission to use the ideas contained in articles published by them: *Journal of Advanced Nursing* ('A participant observation study of power relations between nurses and doctors in a general hospital': 16: 728-35, 1992, reworked in Chapter 5), *Sociology of Health and Illness* ('Women in a women's job: the gendered experience of nurses': 14: 510-27, 1993, reworked in Chapter 6), *Sociology* ('Critical realist ethnography: the case of racism and professionalism in a medical setting': 27: 591-609, 1993, reworked in Chapters 2 and 7), and the *British Journal of Nursing* ('The changing influence of occupational sociology', 2: 1113-19, 1993, reworked in Chapter 4). My reasons for this self-plagiarism are two-fold. Firstly, responses from colleagues to the original works, combined with my own ruminations on them, have led to what I hope is an improvement on the original arguments. Secondly, I believe there is a more general story to be told than can be accommodated in discrete articles. The point of this book is to bring together my interpretation and explanation of the relationship of nursing with medicine into an overarching whole, which I hope will be greater than the sum of the original parts.

As with many an Avebury book, this one is based on my doctoral thesis. I would therefore like to thank the numerous people who helped me with that thesis. However, there are some for whom I would like to make special mention. I wish to thank my initial supervisor, Steve Bruce, whose ascerbic wit did much to sharpen my plodding style. The bulk of supervision was carried out by John Brewer, and I am grateful for the professionalism and erudition he displayed in discharging his task. I also gained invaluable help from my colleagues, Eithne McLaughlin, Robbie McVeigh and Colin Coulter.

My gratitude also goes out to the many nurses who facilitated my research, tolerated my intrusion, or gave up their time to allow me into their confidence.

In 1987, I gave up a perfectly good job as a staff nurse in order to become an impecunious sociology student. This, combined with the advent of offspring, meant that I required more support than I deserved from those close to me. My parents, Joan and Warren Porter, came to my aid without complaint or hesitation. This acknowledgement is small recompense for the kindness they have shown to me.

Finally, I would like to thank Sandra Ryan. Without her intellectual, emotional, moral and financial support, neither the thesis nor the book would have been possible.

List of abbreviations

NHS: National Health Service
UKCC: United Kingdom Central Council for Nursing Health Visiting and Midwifery

ICU: Intensive Care Unit
NDU: Nursing Development Unit

CON: Medical Consultant
D: Domestic Assistant
EN: Enrolled Nurse
JHO: Junior House Officer
MS: Medical Student
REG: Medical Registrar
SHO: Senior House Officer
SN: Staff Nurse
SP: Sam Porter
SR: Ward Sister
T: Nurse Tutor
UC: Unit Co-Ordinator

F: Female
M: Male

Part One

Part One

1 Introduction

Introduction

Nursing is a changing occupation. As we shall see, not least of these changes is the alteration of its relationship with medicine. The purpose of this book is to both describe and explain the nature of this relationship. It will attempt to do so using the tools of sociological analysis. The focus of this analysis will be on two levels, one internal to nursing, and one which locates nursing within the matrix of wider social relations. At an internal level, attention will be upon the specific strategies that have been adopted by 'nursing entrepreneurs' to advance the occupation's position, and the success, or lack of it, that they have met. To this end, concepts like the nursing process, nursing models, primary nursing, and patient advocacy will be introduced, and their import examined.

At the wider social level, nursing is located within the social structures that pertain in the societies in which it exists. Nursing is not immune from the effects of social structures; far from it. One of the central arguments of the book will be that general social factors are crucially important in determining the position of nurses within health care organisations. The effects of three social structures upon the relationship between nursing and medicine will be examined those of patriarchy, racism and capitalism. This is not to say that these were the only social structures that had influence over the social arenas examined in this book. The research for the book having taken place in the north of Ireland, it should come as no surprise to readers that sectarianism had a considerable effect upon relations between health care workers of different ethnic backgrounds. However, as the aim of the book is to construct an analysis that is generalisable over international borders, the specificities of the social context of Ireland are not dealt with in detail.

Patriarchy, racism and capitalism

The most striking sociological fact about nursing is that, in contrast to medicine which has historically been a male-dominated occupation, it is overwhelmingly staffed by women. This has important consequences for the relationship between nursing and medicine. As a women's occupation, nursing has been disadvantaged by its location within a patriarchal society, while medicine has been correspondingly advantaged. On a more optimistic note, any attenuation of the power of patriarchy will have beneficial effects for nurses. One of the arguments of this book will be that changes in the relationship pertaining between nursing and medicine have reflected changes in male-female relations.

Patriarchy is not the only structure that impinges upon the occupational position of nurses. Within the social situation studied, racism was also a pertinent factor in nurse-doctor interactions, in that a significant proportion of doctors belonged to racialised groups (groups to which the ideological category of 'race' has been attributed (Miles 1982)). Ironically, the effects of racism tended to have a countervailing effect to those of patriarchy, in that those that it disadvantaged were members of the medical profession.

In addition to patriarchy and racism, the changing organisation of capitalism, specifically the retrenchment of public health care expenditure and the encroachment of post-Fordist forms of production and consumption, has also affected nursing's relationship with medicine. However, as we shall see, these developments have had contradictory effects upon the occupational position of nursing

The division between internal and external explanations of the occupational position of nursing is to a degree an artificial one. For instance, it is no accident that some of the strategies adopted by nursing entrepreneurs, which involve emphasis on patients as human beings with subjective needs (in contrast to the medical emphasis on patients as scientific objects), mirrors feminist concerns about recognising the importance of personal experience (*cf.* Stanley and Wise 1983). Thus, Hagell argues that:

> nursing, as a discipline, has a distinct knowledge base which is not grounded in empirico-analytical science and its methodology but which stems from the lived experience of nurses as women and as nurses involved in caring relationships with their clients (1989:226).

This radical alteration in the philosophical grounding of health care is an exciting departure which has consequences not only for the relationship between nurse and patient, but also between nurse and doctor. The ramifications of what has been termed 'New Nursing' (Salvage 1990) will be examined.

The organisation of the book

It will be noted that this book is divided into three different parts. Each part has a specific focus. Part One consists of this introduction, and a reflexive account of the methods and methodology adopted in the research.

The purpose of Part Two is to describe the nature of the occupational position of nursing. That can only be fully done by presenting it within its historical context.

4

Thus, Part Two is divided into three chapters. Chapter Three deals with historical relations. It involves secondary analysis of nursing and sociological literature pertaining to nurse-doctor relationships over the last 25 years. Chapter Four examines how nursing entrepreneurs have been influenced by the sociology of professions in their attempts to improve the status of their occupation. Once again, most of the information provided is in the form of a literature review, although the chapter concludes with an examination of how occupational self-concept is taught to nursing students, and how clinical staff interpret their occupational position, using interviews from Suburban Hospital. Chapter Five describes contemporary manifestations of nurse-doctor power relations. Here I use primary ethnographic material. This material consists of two separate groups of data. Firstly, the data that emerged from participant observation of nurses and doctors in an intensive care unit, and secondly, from informal interviews with nurses from a medical unit, a surgical unit and a nursing development unit.

Part Three examines the factors that influence that relationship. The focus is largely on pertinent social structures. Chapters Six to Eight examine how the structures of patriarchy, racism and capitalism impinge upon the occupational relationship that nurses have with their medical colleagues. Chapter Nine qualifies this focus on structure by examining other dynamics that have an effect upon the relationship. Chapter Ten brings the arguments of the book together, and discusses their import.

Theory and practice

The aim of this book is not simply to empirically explicate the position of a specific occupational group. Equal importance is given to the development of adequate theoretical tools to do so. This, at times, requires considerable discursive analysis of theoretical texts. The necessity for such discussion rests on the fact that:

> the many and complex problems of today's world cannot be explained without recourse to *social* theory - a theory which explains why appearances assume the form they do, a theory which reveals the underlying factors, or structure, on which are built the complex realities of everyday life (Crompton and Gubbay: 1977:4, emphasis in original).

Much of my theoretical work centres on Roy Bhaskar's model of critical realism. This is not a free-floating exegesis, but is grounded in the problem at hand, for as Crompton and Gubbay go on to note, 'it must always be remembered that abstract theories stand or fall by the illumination they lend to *empirical* material' (1977:4, emphasis in original). However, it should be said that Bhaskar does not make for easy reading. While I have made efforts here to present his ideas in a more accessible manner than they are presented in the original, some readers may find the theoretical discussions included rather imperspicuous. For those who do not wish to trawl through the rather involved debates contained in the next chapter, in which I explicate my theoretical approach, I include here a brief synopsis of Bhaskar's ideas.

Bhaskar describes his philosophy as 'critical realism'. Inclusion of the word 'realism' comes from the fact that he asserts that there *is* a reality out there that is independent of our observations or thoughts about it. Moreover, Bhaskar argues that reality is not confined to things; it also includes those structures that have effects upon things. Thus, for example, he would argue that the arrangement of iron filings into patterns using a magnet involves two levels of reality. The first and most obvious level is that of the filings themselves, which we can see and touch. However, if we only accepted this level of reality we could not explain why the filings go into the patterns that they do. In order to do so, we must also accept the reality of magnetism which structures the movement and arrangement of those filings. Of course, we can never see or feel magnetism, we can only see or feel its effects. However, for Bhaskar the fact that it has effects is proof of its reality.

Similarly with people, he argues that their actions cannot be explained simply in terms of their individual needs or desires (though he does not wish to deny the importance of those needs and desires). People's actions are not random; their behaviour also has patterns. Therefore, an adequate explanation of human action needs to include identification of the structures that influence those patterns. I choose the word 'influence' carefully. Bhaskar does not seek to portray human beings as automatons who simply respond automatically to the dictates of social structures. Society is an open system, with many structures operating simultaneously, some reinforcing and some contradicting each other. Add to this the psychological structures that we each possess, and firm prediction of the actions of specific individuals becomes impossible; all the social scientist can hope to do is identify the tendencies generated by structures. Nor can social structures be unproblematically equated with natural structures. The most important difference between them is that social structures are not independent of the individuals whose lives they influence, rather they are maintained or transformed by the actions of individuals. Thus, the relationship between structure and action is a two-way process.

The work of the social scientist, according to critical realism, is to identify patterns of social behaviour and ask what social structures must be in existence in order for those patterns to occur. This sort of questioning was first formulated by Immanuel Kant in his critical philosophy, which is one of the reasons why Bhaskar terms his approach '*critical* realism'. The final stage of investigation involves the process of empirically questioning whether the hypotheses formulated can indeed adequately explain the patterned activities observed.

Bhaskar does not see social science as a value-free exercise. By exposing social structures and the restraints and enablements that they impose upon our freedom to act in our own interests, it provides us with knowledge that can be used in attempts to improve the structural organisation of society. In this particular case, it is hoped that, by demonstrating the salience of social structures to the occupational position of nursing, the following account will persuade readers that sole concentration on internal professional dynamics will not be sufficient to deliver the autonomy that many nurses aspire to.

Theory versus empiricism

What, it might be asked, is the point of applying these fairly esoteric philosophical ideas to the issue of nursing's relationship with medicine? Does such an approach have any merit in adding to our knowledge of the social world? Two lines of response could be made to such queries. First would be the claim that it is helpful to nurses to be aware of the broader social context of their occupational position. However, I will leave discussion of the issue until the concluding chapter of the book. What I wish to do here is briefly outline the ways in which the approach taken here might contribute to sociological knowledge *per se*. It is almost a truism that sociology has been characterised by dichotomous interpretations as to its appropriate focus. However, in recent years, the art of synthesis has increasingly come to the fore within the discipline. One of the aims of this book is to contribute to the efforts of sociologists attempting to transcend intellectual divisions.

A significant fissure within sociology, identified by Bulmer (1989), is the divide amongst its practitioners between theoretical and substantive concerns. Bulmer complains that much recent sociological work concentrates exclusively on matters theoretical, treating the need for empirical information about the social world in a cavalier fashion.

While much of this book is devoted to theoretical discussion, I have made a conscious effort to ensure that that discussion remains in contact with the substantive issue at hand; that apparently esoteric theories are marshalled to improve understanding of the empirical phenomena that are identified. In doing so, I hope to demonstrate that the divide between theory and empirical investigation is not a necessary one, indeed, that neither can provide adequate knowledge on its own (Crompton and Gubbay 1977).

Science versus interpretation

Another aim of the book is to overcome the hoary dichotomy between positivism and interpretive approaches that has bedevilled sociological thought almost since its outset. By using critical realism, I hope to demonstrate the possibility of naturalism in the human sciences (to use Bhaskar's (1989b) phrase,[1] while at the same time taking account of the interpretive critique of previous scientistic constructions of social knowledge. As I have noted above, critical realism entails the rejection of the positivist assumption that the identification of constant conjunctions is the aim of natural science, and should be the aim of social science. Instead, it is argued that both the natural and social worlds are open systems, and as a consequence the aim of science is to identify tendencies generated by structures, rather than invariant causal relationships.

In human sciences, matters are further complicated by the fact that individuals are reflexive. The effects of social structures are therefore mediated through the psyches of agents. Nevertheless, it is possible both to identify structures and the influences that those structures have upon human behaviour. This is not to reify social structures; critical realism accepts that another limitation on naturalism is the fact that social structures are dependent upon phenomena for their existence, in that it is the actions of human agents that either reproduce or transform them.

Structure versus action

Another dichotomy that has troubled sociology is that between structure and agency. As will be noted in Chapter Two, there have been numerous attempts to resolve this problem. I have chosen critical realism for two reasons. Firstly because it gives powerful emphasis to the importance of social structures, an importance that has often been forgotten in recent sociological work. The recent postmodern turn in social thought has led to a suspicion of 'totalising discourses' which attempt to explain all social life within the confines of an overarching model. On these grounds, Marxism has been rejected by many because of its perceived economic reductionism. Critical realism takes cognisance of this criticism through its acceptance that there is no single structure governing social life. However, it avoids the error of swinging to the other extreme of portraying social life as free-floating voluntarism on the part of isolated individuals.

This closely relates to the second strength of critical realism to which I was attracted, namely that it is not a disinterested philosophical position. Rather, it is constructed as a component part of the project of human emancipation. As such, it is an attempt to redeem the aspirations of the Enlightenment.

The dangers of eclecticism

It will be seen from the discussion above, that in attempting to address fundamental issues which have troubled sociology for so long, I am setting myself a very tall order. To make matters worse, my substantive focus is equally, if not more, wide ranging. One of the characteristics of the book is that it ranges over a considerable number of the sub-disciplines which make up the body of sociological knowledge. Thus, I utilise, amongst others, the sociology of gender, 'race', organisations and occupational culture, to say nothing of to say nothing of political economy and nursing knowledge, in order to elucidate the nature of nursing's relationship with medicine. While there is considerable danger of my being a jack of all trades and master of none, I would argue that there are good reasons for this eclecticism.

While the expansion of sociology has inevitably entailed specialisation, it is my contention that the division of the discipline into a myriad of self-contained discourses has entailed the compromising of holistic social understanding. To attempt to explain the social lives of people in terms of a single explanatory approach is to do violence to social reality. The lives of women cannot be fully understood without knowledge of the economic structures within which they work; the experience of black people cannot be understood without taking into account their gendered position. The aim of this book was to develop a rounded approach to the occupational position of nurses; in doing so it is necessary to cast a wide net. It is hoped that such an approach will demonstrate both the benefit and viability of a synthesising approach to knowledge of the social world.

Orientation to time and space

While this book is about nursing, it is not about nursing just anywhere; it is specifically located in time and space. Empirical information was gained from the qualitative study of nurses working in three institutions in the north of Ireland between 1989 and 1993.

Nursing in the north of Ireland is organised along similar lines to nursing in Britain. Professional control rests with the United Kingdom Central Council for Nursing, Midwifery and Health Visiting (UKCC). As with Scotland, Wales and England, there is an executive 'National' Board for the area, which formulates and arranges courses and examinations on behalf of the UKCC.

As in Britain, most health care is provided through the National Health Service (NHS), although there are two private hospitals in the region. All of the nurses involved in this study worked for the NHS. While the NHS in the north of Ireland has been subjected to the same reforms as its counterpart in Britain during the 1980s and 1990s, the pace of change has been much slower. The reason for this was that the proconsuls governing the area have consistently taken a 'wetter' line in relation to the welfare state than their colleagues in Westminster. This tardiness in the application of Thatcherite principles meant that, during the period when I conducted research by participant observation in 1989 and 1990, the Salmon system of management, with its nursing line management structures, was extant in the hospital I was working in. Similarly, in 1992 and 1993, while I was conducting interviews in another hospital, that hospital had yet to become a self-governing trust.

However, as far as nursing education is concerned, the peculiarities of the north of Ireland lie in the opposite direction, with the National Board for Nursing, Midwifery, and Health Visiting for Northern Ireland (National Board) enthusiastically adopting the reforms set out by the UKCC. In 1987, the UKCC published its final proposals for the 'Project 2000' reforms of nursing education. Proposed was the scrapping of two-tier training, and its replacement by a single level of registered nurse. Training would consist of an 18-month common foundation programme, followed by a further 18 months of specialist training. Considerably more emphasis was to be put on academic work. Greater time was to be spent on lectures, and when students were in the clinical area they were to be supernumerary to staffing establishments.[2] The aim of the reforms was to enable nurses to become 'knowledgeable doers'.

In May 1988, the Secretary of State for Social Services, John Moore accepted most of the Council's proposals, and the stage was set for implementation. In response, steering committees were set up by the Department of Health and Social Services (NI), and by the National Board. The conclusion that these committees came to was

9

that the most appropriate route to implementation in the north of Ireland was by the 'big bang' approach (Slevin 1989), which entailed the colleges of nursing in the region commencing the Project 2000 Common Foundation Programme *en masse* between October 1990 and March 1991. The students examined in this book belonged to the last cohort of the traditional training programme.

Implementation of Project 2000 was envisaged as only stage one of nursing education reforms. The long-term strategy was full integration with the University sector as soon as possible after the year 2000 (National Board 1989). However, things have moved much faster than the National Board anticipated. In 1992, a working party convened by the Department of Health and Social Services (NI) and the Department of Health for Northern Ireland (1992) proposed that integration should occur in 1995. Preparations for this are now well underway.

There have also been developments in relation to the nurse-patient relationship. The Government's *Charter for Patients and Clients* now requires that each patient is allocated a named nurse (Northern Ireland Health and Personal Social Services 1992). This is consonant with the movement towards primary nursing, the system whereby one nurse is specifically responsible for the care of a small group of patients, which has been enthusiastically promoted in the region by the Northern Ireland Primary Nursing Network (Mullholland and Griffiths 1991).

Another facet of New Nursing that had been adopted by one of the hospitals where this research took place, was the inauguration of a Nursing Development Unit (NDU). NDUs are defined by Black as:

> a team of nurses ... who have as their prime purpose the development of nursing practice. Underpinning the initiative is the belief that nurses themselves are well placed to introduce innovations and that changes in nursing practice can benefit patients (1992:2).

It can be seen that nurses in the north of Ireland are deeply involved in attempts to alter the role and standing of nursing. As such, they provide an appropriate focus for research into the occupational position of nursing and its relation to medicine.

Sic men

I wish to conclude this introduction with a brief note on language. Throughout the book, I endeavour to use non-sexist language. However, on numerous occasions, the sources that I cite do not. Initially, I appended a 'sic' to each instance of sexist language. However, this device appeared cumbersome, and, so it seemed to me, gave the book an air of sanctimoneous political correctness. Therefore, I have decided on the more economical tactic of stating at the outset my awareness and disapproval of the previously prevalent practice of excising women from sociological discourse, while leaving the texts I quote in their original without comment.

Notes

1. There is some confusion in the term 'naturalism'. It has been used by some qualitative methodologists to denote the study of the social world in its 'natural' state (Hammersley and Atkinson 1983), rather than through the use of artificial, 'scientific' methods. However, Bhaskar is using the term in the sense that it has been given within the discourse of the philosophy of science, a sense that is almost diametrically opposed to that of the qualitative methodologists. Here, the possibility of naturalism is taken to mean the extent to which society can be studied in the same way as nature.

2. The attainment of supernumerary status was an important goal. Melia (1987) observed that the system of learning which predominantly located students as clinical-based apprentices meant that the theoretical knowledge that they gained from their limited sojourns in college was quickly drowned by the exigencies of work.

2 Method and methodology

Introduction

This chapter is divided into three broad sections. Each section concerns a different moment in the process of 'reflexivity'; a process which entails, in the words of Alvin Gouldner's Yeatsian allusion, researchers casting 'a cold eye on their own doings' (1971:488).

The chapter commences with a discussion of the theoretical principles upon which my research was conducted, with particular reference to the recent debate around what Brewer (1994) has termed the 'ethnographic critique of ethnography'. The purpose of this discussion is to satisfy one of the criteria that Brewer identifies as good ethnographic practice; that ethnographers should 'identify the theoretical framework they are operating within, and the broader values and commitments ... they bring to their work' (1994:235). My response to the problems raised by the ethnographic critique of ethnography is to frame my work around the theoretical model of critical realism.

Having set out my methodological wares, I then move on to another aspect of ethnographic reflexivity, emphasised by Hammersley and Atkinson (1983). This involves description and reflection upon the import of the methods used in the research and the context within which the research was conducted.

Building upon this discussion, I use the final section to reflect on how personal factors specific to my own biography may have affected my research, and the results gleaned from it. In doing so, I am following the injunction of Aldridge, who argues that, rather than excising their experiences from the research, research account writers 'should instead use these experiences analytically' (1993:64).

The ethnographic critique of ethnography

In the wake of general acceptance of the role of qualitative methods within sociology, recent criticisms of ethnography have tended to emanate from sympathetic, rather than ideologically opposed, commentators. This, however, does not make their observations any the less telling.

While attention was fixed on the motes in the sociological eye of positivism, the moral entrepreneurs of ethnography could afford to gloss over the inevitable inconsistencies within their own philosophy. However, with the battle won, and ethnography accepted into mainstream sociological method, its own optical beams are coming increasingly under scrutiny.

One of the most significant interventions of late has been that of Martyn Hammersley.[1] I propose here to engage with the ideas contained in two of his papers: 'What's wrong with ethnography?' (1990) and 'Ethnography and realism' (in Hammersley 1992). I will argue that one possible solution to the problems posed is the adoption of critical realism as an underlabouring philosophy for ethnographic research.

What's wrong with ethnography?

Hammersley's (1990) argument centres around the epistemological claims that are made for ethnography. In particular, he focuses on the connection between ethnographic description and social theory, examining four alternative rationales for their relationship. The basic assumption behind these rationales is that ethnography is capable of providing a distinctive type of description, one which is pregnant with theoretical import. Hammersley terms this construct 'theoretical description'.

The first variant of theoretical description that Hammersley addresses is that of 'insightful description'. This involves the claim that ethnographic descriptions can present phenomena in new and revealing ways. The most spectacular examples of this approach can be seen in Everett Hughes's (1971) and Erving Goffman's (1968) use of analogies and metaphors to reinterpret various social phenomena. Despite such prestigious parentage, Hammersley argues that insightful description is flawed because it cannot be subjected to adequate evaluation. Instead, it tends to be judged according to its novelty, or its aesthetic or political appeal. This immunity from rigorous testing makes such an approach less than convincing.

Abstracted empiricism

Hammersley calls the second rationale 'theory as the description of social microcosms'. Advocates of this approach contend that universal social processes are to be identified through the description of particular events. In response, Hammersley questions the logical possibility of description (relating to particulars) being able to generate theory (relating to universals).

Hammersley's anti-inductivist critique echoes C. Wright Mills's assault on 'abstracted empiricism'. Mills contended that the assumption that an integrated

13

social science could be constructed by bringing together the results of numerous small investigations was inadequate. He argued that:

> The problems of social science are stated in terms of conceptions that usually relate to social-historical structures. If we take such problems as real, then it does seem foolish to undertake any detailed studies of smaller-scale areas before we have good reason to believe that, whatever the results, they will permit us to draw inferences useful in solving or clarifying problems of structural significance (1970:77).

The advancement of knowledge depends upon a combination of theory and investigation (Merton 1968). Moreover, within the relationship, theory can claim at least temporal priority. Without what Heidegger (1962) termed 'pre-understandings', identification or analysis of situations would be impossible. It behoves social investigators to make the pre-understandings under which they labour explicit to both themselves and their readers.

Hammersley charges ethnographers with a commitment to what he calls the 'reproduction model of research', which claims to be able to describe the social world as it really is. He observes that truth underdetermines descriptions and that other values and concerns also play a role in their production. Acceptance of the validity of the reproduction model leads to a failure to make explicit the theoretical assumptions and values upon which research is predicated.

Methodological individualism

The above quotation from Mills indicates another assumption that is often implicit in the 'social microcosm' approach, that of methodological individualism: 'the doctrine that all social phenomena ... are in principle explicable in ways that only involve individuals - their properties, their goals, their beliefs and their actions' (Elster 1985:5). This position is explicitly adopted by micro-sociological theorists such as Collins, who argues that social structures are merely aggregates of micro-events, bereft of causal power:

> Social patterns, institutions, and organizations are only abstractions from the behavior of individuals and summaries of the distribution of different microbehaviors in time and space. These abstractions and summaries do not *do* anything (1981:989, emphasis in original).

It would, of course, be a travesty to unproblematically equate micro-sociology with methodological individualism. Knorr-Cetina (1988), for example, explicitly rejects methodological individualism, arguing that neither individual psychologies nor subjective intentions can provide an elementary basis for social reality. Nevertheless, her concept of 'methodological situationalism', while giving analytic priority to the social situation of individuals, rather than to the individuals themselves, still contains the assumption that macro-phenomena ultimately refer to micro-scale

14

ontological

transactions; that structures consist of 'interrelationships between micro-episodes' (Knorr-Cetina 1988:39).

The relationship between structure and action is not discussed by Hammersley here. However, given the fundamental importance of this antinomy (Mouzelis 1993), it is one of the theoretical assumptions that the ethnographer is required to make explicit if the naiveté of the reproduction model is to be avoided.

Analytic description

Hammersley accepts that the third variant, 'analytic description', is methodologically more conventional than the previous two. Rather than claiming that description is capable of generating theory, this model presents description as an empirical tool for the application and modification of theory.

Once again, however, Hammersley questions the amenability of this form of ethnography to testing. He points out that even advocates of this approach admit that one study, because it is only a single case, cannot itself provide a powerful test of theory (McCall and Simmons 1969). Therefore testing comes through the comparison of a number of analytic descriptions. Herein lies the problem. Because ethnographic studies are largely formulated in terms of the subject being examined rather than the theory being tested, the inherent variations in description make comparison of cases well nigh impossible. If it is accepted that the purpose of ethnography is to empirically test social theory, then it would seem a logical corollary that ethnographic research should primarily focus on the theoretical problem at hand rather than on the substantive subject matter.

Critical cases

The final variation of theoretical description, what Hammersley calls 'ethnography as developing theory through the study of critical cases', attempts to surmount this problem by consciously selecting cases through reference to the theoretical issues being addressed.

However, while this variant overcomes Hammersley's objections to the previous construct, he remains unhappy with its methodological bases, which he identifies as grounded theory and analytic induction. Grounded theory is criticised because of the ambiguity of its role. It is unclear whether grounded theory was designed to develop theory or also to test it. The use of analytic induction by ethnographers is also seen by Hammersley as inappropriate because of what he sees as the scientistic assumptions that are embedded in it, most notably its affinity with the hypothetico-deductive method. Because ethnography rejects deterministic causation, amenable to hypothetico-deductivist verification (or falsification), Hammersley argues that it can only provide explanations in terms of teleology or ideal type. This level of explanation, he contends, is no different from that employed in everyday life.

It is in Hammersley's criticisms of this variant of ethnography that I part company with him. As Stanley (1990) observes, his focus on ethnography is unfairly narrow. The problems he alludes to are pertinent to all types of social research. Indeed,

15

Hammersley himself (Hammersley and Atkinson 1983) has previously laid the same charge of similarity to everyday explanations at the door of the experimental method. It is ironic, then, that Hammersley now appears to be arguing that social analysts cannot rise above everyday perspectives because they cannot accept the ontology of deterministic laws or the epistemology of the experimental method. Nevertheless, his criticisms do underline the obligation of investigators to address the level of explanation that their work can support.

From the above discussion we can distil a number of problems that face the aspiring ethnographer:

1 There is a need to make apparent the assumptions and values that underlie a particular investigation.

2 There is a need to focus empirical research on the theoretical issues that it is designed to illuminate.

3 There is a need to make explicit the ontological status ascribed to social structures.

4 There is a need to examine the explanatory status of a methodology which rejects determinism.

The pertinence of critical realism

It is my contention that the use of Roy Bhaskar's critical realism is one way to solve these problems. Critical realism is an attempt to explain the relationship of social structure and human action. It rejects both individualist voluntarism, and collectivist reification of social entities. Instead, it argues that:

> the existence of social structure is a necessary condition for any human activity. Society provides the means, media, rules and resources for everything we do ... It is the unmotivated condition for all our motivated productions. We do not create society - the error of voluntarism. But these structures which pre-exist us are only reproduced or transformed in our everyday activities; thus society does not exist independently of human agency - the error of reification. The social world is reproduced and transformed in daily life (1989a:3-4).

This position echoes the Marxian dictum that 'Men make their own history, but not spontaneously, under conditions they have chosen for themselves; rather on terms immediately existing, given and handed down to them' (Marx 1983:287).

According to critical realism, social phenomena are the result of a plurality of structures (Bhaskar 1989a). These structures are, of course, unperceivable. They cannot, therefore, be identified except through examination of their effects. Nor indeed, can they exist independently of them (Bhaskar 1989b). However, it is the very existence of these effects that demonstrate the reality of structures. Bhaskar argues that there are two criteria for the ascription of reality: perceptual and causal. The requirement of the latter criterion is the ability of an entity to bring about changes in material things. The mistake of anti-naturalists such as Winch (1958) is to assume that mechanisms have to be perceivable to be real. This yardstick of reality would exclude such natural forces as magnetism and gravity. In the last instance, to be is not to be directly perceived but to be able to do (Bhaskar 1978). Because social structures constrain and enable human actions, they satisfy the causal criterion of reality.

Social analysis consists of synthetic *a priori* production of hypotheses about the nature of structures, and subsequent testing of them through empirical examination of their effects. Structures are hypothetically identified through the use of transcendental questions, which involve asking what must be the case for a certain human activity to be possible.

Critical realism and the ethnographic critique

Thus far, the first three issues arising from Hammersley's critique have been addressed. The basic theoretical assumption of critical realism is that human action is enabled and constrained by social structures, but that action, in turn, reproduces or transforms those structures. Acceptance of the reality of social structures entails the rejection of methodological individualism as a sufficient mode of explanation. Similarly, methodological situationalism is seen as providing too weak a conception of structure.

Theoretical analysis of the nature of structures is an essential prerequisite to the understanding of social phenomena. In turn, theories about the nature of social structures and their effects upon human action need to be empirically tested. This testing is complicated by the fact that the subject matter of social science is conceptual. This limits the explanatory power of quantitative measurement. As Bhaskar puts it: 'meanings cannot be measured, only understood' (1989b:46). Thus there is a need for the qualitative testing of hypotheses about the nature and effects of generative structures upon human action and vice versa. It is at this stage that ethnographic techniques can play a role. The purpose of ethnographic investigation here is not to idiographically illuminate small scale social events, but to use examination of human agency to shed light on the relationship between agency and structure. It is therefore necessary to explicitly focus research on the effects of the structural phenomena that are thought to be involved. This concentration on structures, rather than events *sui generis*, facilitates comparative testing of conclusions drawn.

Textual construction

It has to be conceded that the exposing of prior theoretical assumptions, while it entails rejection of naive realist pretentions, does not exhaust the thorny problem of representation. The issue is not simply how the researcher perceives the data, it is also how s\he portrays it. Betwixt interaction and publication, data is subjected to

17

several stages of translation and transcription (Atkinson 1990). This process involves manipulation of the data so that it fits with the arguments that are being promulgated (Williams 1990) The great danger here is that the events being described will be 'subverted by the transcending stories in which they are cast' (Crapanzano 1986:76). Given the transcendental aspects of critical realism, it would seem that it is especially prone to this error. Nevertheless, I would argue that recognition that critical realist ethnography, as any other, is not written in a neutral descriptive language does not lead to the relativist view that regards every ethnography as an invention of its author (*cf.* Clifford 1986). Rather, I would concur with Atkinson (1990) that awareness of the processes by which our understandings are fashioned can only strengthen our critical reflection.

Causes as tendencies

I now turn to the fourth problem: Hammersley argues that because ethnographers do not accept the existence of deterministic social laws, the theories they generate can be nothing more than teleological or ideal typical. He notes that it is only on the assumption 'that there are scientific laws of human social life (and deterministic rather than probabilistic ones at that) ... that reconstruction of theory in the face of conflicting evidence makes any sense' (1990: 604-5). Implicit in Hammersley's argument is the assumption that, because of the reflexivity of the human subject, it cannot be studied in the same manner as the natural object, which, being unreflexive, is governed by deterministic laws. According to critical realism, such a dichotomy is false. Bhaskar argues that the belief that deterministic laws can be identified through the study of constant conjunctions,[2] occurring within the artificially enclosed environment of the experiment, fails to recognise the reality of both the social and natural worlds; namely that they are open systems. He argues that in open systems, constant conjunctions do not pertain. Therefore,

> causal laws must be analysed as the tendencies of things, which may be possessed unexercised and exercised unrealised, just as they may of course be realised unperceived ... Thus in citing a law one is ... not making a claim about the actual outcome (which will in general be co-determined by the activity of other mechanisms) (1989b: 9-10).

The aim of science, both natural and social, therefore, becomes the identification of the structures and mechanisms which generate tendencies in the behaviour of phenomena. In the case of humans, these phenomena are attitudes and actions. While the reflexive nature of humanity may entail qualitative differences between methods of studying people and other phenomena, this does not mean that we are forced to choose between crude positivism and the abandonment of any nomothetic pretentions whatsoever.

To summarise, ethnographic techniques can be used within the model of critical realism to investigate the nature of generative structures through examination of social phenomena. While such a use of ethnographic techniques involves stripping ethnography of much of its epistemological baggage, it has the merit of surmounting many of the objections to that epistemology posed by Hammersley. Put another way, this approach abandons the *methodology* normally associated with ethnography, but continues to use ethnographic methods in data analysis (for further explication of the articulation between ethnography as method and as methodology, see Brewer 1994).

Critical realism is, of course, not the only attempt to come to terms with the complex relationship between structure and agency. Notable alternatives include Berger and Luckmann's (1971) thesis on the social construction of reality, Giddens' (1984) structuration theory, and the work of Rom Harré (1979). Bhaskar (1989b) criticises the former model for its attempt to dialectically relate structure and action as two moments of the same process, which results in a failure to identify the radical differences between them. Structuration theory is closer to critical realism. However, an important difference lies in interpretation of the significance of structure. While structuration theory emphasises the autonomy of social actors, critical realism underlines the pre-existence of social forms, thus giving structure a stronger ontological grounding (Bhaskar 1983). This emphasis on structure provides a useful antidote to the methodological individualist tendencies of much ethnography. For similar reasons, I did not select Harré's work as the theoretical foundation for this study. While Harré seems to accept the existence of social structures, he is rather dubious about our ability to understand them. In his own words, 'we enter what is plainly a theatre, but we have to guess what play is being performed' (1979:139). Contrary to this position, one of the contentions of this book is that social structures are epistemologically amenable.

Critical versus subtle realism

Critical realism has a good deal in common with Hammersley's (1992) prescription for a 'subtle realism' in ethnography. While he rejects radical constructivism because of the relativist dead-end that it entails, Hammersley argues that naive realism is equally unacceptable because it assumes the possibility of direct contact with reality; contact which will provide certain knowledge of its nature. In other words, contrary to the tenets of the reproduction model of research, subtle realism includes the assumption that knowledge cannot be directly read off from being. Representation of reality will differ according to the point of view adopted. Bhaskar (1991) approaches this problem from the other end, arguing that statements about being cannot be reduced to statements about knowledge. Both realisms, therefore, contain the stricture that knowledge should not be conflated with existence.

The most significant fissure between subtle and critical realism lies in how evaluation of the attitudes and actions of ethnographic subjects is regarded.

Hammersley (1992) argues that the aim of ethnography should be to understand the perspectives of others rather than to judge them. He advises that ethnographers should suspend any beliefs that conflict with those being described in order to avoid misunderstanding. By contrast, Bhaskar (1989a) is explicit in his assertion that critical realism logically entails evaluation. His position could be described as one of 'moral realism', the assumption that fact and value cannot be neatly distinguished and that moral judgements are as amenable to rational argumentation as descriptive statements (Eagleton 1991). Indeed, his position is stronger than this; he regards critical evaluation of structures and of their effects upon human ideology and agency as imperative.

This disagreement over evaluation is associated with differing conceptions about the role of social analysis. Hammersley takes the view that sociology is largely insulated from its subject matter: 'for the most part reality is independent of the claims that social researchers make about it' (1992:51). Conversely, Bhaskar (1989a) contends that social theory and social reality are causally interdependent. Because social analysis may have practical consequences in society, the evaluation that analysts put upon specific social phenomena is crucial.

There are dangers in adopting either side in this controversy. While it is important to realise that 'the social world may be opaque to the social agents upon whom it depends' (Bhaskar 1989a:4), distinguishing between clarity and opacity is problematic, given that analysts themselves cannot have direct contact with the reality of social structures. It has been argued that acceptance of the interpretations of social actors being studied avoids the danger of legislating social structure by fiat (Dingwall 1977). However, while there may be difficulties in gaining knowledge of structures, in that they can only be identified through examination of the actions and interpretations of individuals, this does not mean that they do not exist. By ignoring the potentially constraining nature of social structures, commentators are in danger of giving consent, through silence, to their oppressive effects.

Consider, for example, an ethnographic study of British soldiers (Hockey 1986), part of which involves an account of combat duty in rural Ireland (offensively described as 'bandit country'). While the soldiers' everyday lives in 'XMG' are lavishly portrayed, there is no discussion at all as to why they are there in the first place. More generally, while the study provides us with ample evidence that the outlook of British soldiers is largely mediated through sexist frames of reference, it makes little attempt to critically analyse this phenomenon, beyond portraying it as part of the aggressive masculinity that is seen as necessary for military effectiveness. Nor was it the aim of the author to make such an attempt. He is quite clear about the scope of his research, which involved stressing 'the importance of interpreting the behaviour of people *in terms of their subjectively intended meanings*' (Hockey 1986:10, my emphasis).

Exclusive concentration on, and uncritical acceptance of, subjects' own accounts is the Achilles heel of phenomenological ethnography. It is the *reductio ad absurdum* of the valid hermeneutic point that the social world cannot be fully understood without taking account of the interpretations of the social actors in it. Understanding actors' viewpoints may be a necessary condition for social knowledge, but it is not a sufficient one. The ontological assumption that individual interactions and interpretations are ultimately all there are leads to analytic superficiality. As Marx pithily remarked, 'all science would be superfluous if the outward appearances and essences of things directly coincided' (1966:817).

Underlabouring philosophy

The utility of theoretical constructs can only be assessed through their application to concrete examples. The usefulness claimed by critical realism rests on its ability to act as an 'underlabouring' philosophy for social science (Bhaskar 1989a). The Lockean conception of underlabouring involves 'clearing the ground a little, and removing some of the rubbish that lies in the way of knowledge' (Locke 1894:14), so that the builders of science can go about their task less encumbered. Whether this exercise in ideological refuse disposal has been successful will be judged according to its utility in helping us to understand specific aspects of the social world with greater clarity. One of the primary tasks of this book is to use the social dynamics of nurse-doctor relations as a test case, to see if critical realism can provide an adequate explanation for the interactions observed.

However, before going any further, I am obliged to engage with a criticism which models of the social world associated with underlabouring theory and realism have been subjected to.

There are two objections here. First, it is posited that to adopt a realist position is to deny the situational specificity of social life. Second, the building of 'grand narratives' is associated with patriarchal values. These two points are combined in Williams's application to ethnography of Stanley's (1987) 'reverse archaeology's biographical technique:

> I insist on producing a knowledge that assumes I am part of the world I study. To take this position is to move away from presenting knowledge only from the standpoint of 'the rulers' - the patriarchal forms of contemporary experience ... to move away from only knowing ourselves through the ideas and concepts of patriarchy ... This is part of what I am trying to do ... in taking a 'reverse archaeology approach' to understanding the field, to render the field as problematic and complex, rather than simply stripping away layers of knowledge as 'debris' which prevents us from seeing the real X or Y beneath (Williams 1990:18).

In elucidating her concept of reverse archaeology, Stanley (1987) uses the metaphor of the kaleidoscope. In doing so, she goes beyond the traditional perspectivist position that different observers will have different perspectives of a particular phenomenon. She argues that the same observer will perceive constantly changing patterns in the social relations they observe. She links this assertion of the indeterminacy of knowledge with feminist methodology.

Stanley's position is consonant with the recent postmodern 'turn' in feminist theorising, which criticises Enlightenment rationalism for its intrinsic patriarchal nature, and its denial of feminine experience. Thus, for example, Hekman argues:

> Feminists have defined what the postmoderns call 'logocentrism' as an inherently masculine mode of thought. Thus, like the postmoderns, they challenge the Enlightenment's concepts of truth and rationality. Although the other dichotomies that inform the postmodern position are important, the rational\irrational dualism is particularly fundamental to the postmodern attack on logocentrism and the connection between that attack and contemporary feminism (1990:11).

As a man writing about the experiences of a group dominated by women, using a model which is firmly placed within neo-Enlightenment thought, it is incumbent upon me to be sensitive to such criticisms, and to justify my position.

Not all feminist theorists have adopted a postmodern position. Johnson (1993) argues that the attack made by some feminists on the Enlightenment is the result of a misconstrual of its essential meaning as an unfinished cultural project. While she endorses feminist critiques of the Enlightenment which seek to unmask the ways in which Western reason have been used to embody the norms of a male-dominated culture, she argues that this does not warrant the radical separation of contemporary feminism from the influence of Enlightenment thinking. Instead, she argues that feminism should be viewed as taking the Enlightenment project a stage further:

> Enlightenment means only a commitment to an ongoing critique of prejudice and to the historical production of a self-legislating humanity. This commitment which has threaded its way through the intellectual trajectory of modernity exists as a living, dynamic aspiration which is fundamentally irreducible to any one single formulation. So it seems that the acknowledgement of feminism's own Enlightenment character by no means signifies its assimilation to any pre-existing goals and perspectives. On the contrary, feminism's current critique of Enlightenment formulations appears as another vital episode in the unfolding of the Enlightenment project itself. Feminism's discovery of the prejudices built into the various articulations of this project is nothing more than an extension and clarification of the meaning of the Enlightenment (1993:4).

A similar position is taken by Bauman, who argues that, despite its failures, the potential of modernity remains untapped, and its promise needs to be redeemed. This redemption will require that 'the unbreakable link between the enhancement of person-oriented values [of autonomy, self-perfection and authenticity] and the construction of the rational society is once more brought into relief and made visible' (1987:191).

On such an account, rationality, rather than being a tool for patriarchy, is conceived as the bedrock of liberatory praxis, for women just as much as for the rest of humanity. Thus, rather than presenting knowledge from the standpoint of 'the rulers', critical realism asserts:

> that the possibility of a scientific *critique* of lay ... ideas, grounded in explanatory practices based on respect for the authenticity and epistemic significance of those ideas, affords to the human sciences an essential emancipatory impulse (Bhaskar 1989a:89, emphasis in original).

As part of this process, recognition of the influence of structures is essential, because it is only through the construction of explanatory theories which elucidate structures of oppression, and the possibility of their transformation by women and men, that human emancipation is possible.[4]

This is not to say that critical realism claims to stand above the world it studies. Rather, 'it is part of the very process it describes ... Hence continuing self-reflexive auto-critique is the *sine qua non* of any critical explanatory theory' (Bhaskar 1989a:114).

Before engaging in a reflexive explication of the methods that I used in this research, and the contingencies that impinged upon my efforts, I wish to briefly address a final issue related to the reverse archaeology position, namely the assertion that attempts to uncover reality tend to deny the problematic and complex nature of the field under study. This argument has considerable force; reducing the contingencies of social life to the duality of social structures and individual agents that is implied in the critical realist model inevitably entails over-simplification. While I believe that the importance of this duality justifies critical realism's concentration on it as a primary analytic category, I have to concede that it is not the whole story. To counter-balance this theoretical bias, Chapter Four will discuss how the efforts of nursing entrepreneurs have affected the general position of nursing, and Chapter Nine will involve a multi-layered analysis of the social situation that nurses and doctors work in, emphasising its complexity.

Reflections on method and context

In this section, I wish to outline the practicalities of my research, and to discuss how these affected the sort of information that I was able to gather. As I noted in the introduction, this report of the methods and context of my research will be reflexively framed. As Hammersley and Atkinson note, it is a prerequisite of adequate social research for the researcher 'to recognize that we are part of the social world we study ... This is not a matter of methodological commitment, it is an existential fact' (1983:14-15).

The two primary research methods used were participant observation and informal interviews.

The participant observer role that I took was that of staff nurse in an intensive care unit (ICU) in a hospital located in the north of Ireland. I gained this role by the simple expediency of applying for a temporary staff nurse's position, and being accepted. I had no choice in the type of unit that I worked in, the ICU being the only area requiring temporary staff at that juncture. On completing my initial three month contract, I was then invited to join the 'bank nurse' list. This meant that during holidays, and other periods of staff shortage, I was contacted and asked to work on the unit.

I chose an urban general hospital (henceforth referred to as the Metropolitan Hospital) to apply to, both because I hoped that the size and urban location of the hospital would mean that local idiosyncrasies would be minimised, thus enhancing the external validity of the research, and because it was located within manageable commuting distance from my home.

This is not to deny that there were specificities unique to this institution. It was one of two major hospitals in the city where it was located. The Metropolitan Hospital started its existence as a workhouse, was now housed in a modern building. By contrast, the other major hospital was originally a voluntary hospital, with much of its Victorian buildings extant. Their different histories gave these two institutions significantly different cultures, in that the Metropolitan Hospital had a culture of modernity and innovation, while the other hospital's culture emphasised tradition and established status.

During this period, I not only observed, but also conducted short informal interviews with the people I was working with.

My method was largely, but not entirely, overt. While I was quite open about the fact that I was examining interaction between nurses and doctors, I did not emphasise that I was interested in how this related to issues such as racism. The reason for my economy with the truth was that I felt that by highlighting these issues, I would be in danger of driving their manifestation underground. For example, if white nurses who held racist beliefs were aware that one of my primary concerns was racism towards black doctors, then they would be less likely to express their racism in interactions observed by me. I was less coy with nurses about my interest in the issue of sexism. I felt able to be more open because, within female nursing discourse, this issue was not taboo. Indeed, it was relatively frequently alluded to without my encouragement.

I found little resistance from those I was working with to my carrying out research into inter-occupational interactions. The reasons for this were probably different for nurses and doctors. Within nursing culture, research is increasingly valued, and is fairly commonplace (Abdellah and Levine 1979; Wilson-Barnett and Robinson 1989). To the nurses on the unit, my research was seen as unremarkable. As far as doctors were concerned, they took little interest. This was partially due to disdain on the part of some, but it also reflected the fact that I was far more interested in the interpretations of nurses, and as a consequence my prying was largely directed towards them, rather than their medical colleagues.

When applying for the job of staff nurse, I did not inform the hospital's management that I was going to conduct research. My reason for this was that I had previously applied to another hospital in the area, admitting my research interest, and was informed that I could come in and act as participant observer on an unpaid basis. My impecunious situation at the time meant that unwaged research was a luxury that I could not afford. I did not see any medico-ethical problems in this omission, in that I did not feel that my research was of a nature that would compromise patients' welfare. My opinion was reinforced by the attitudes of those managers whom I initially contacted. They had considered my research proposal, and had come to the conclusion that it did not require validation from an ethics committee. Nor did they see any potential violation of staffs' rights, as long as I maintained their anonymity.

Working in an intensive care unit facilitated observation. Firstly, six out of the eight beds in the unit were situated in one room. As a consequence, a large proportion of staff activity was easily observable. Secondly, the nature of intensive care nursing, with its high nurse-patient ratio, meant that I had time to observe and record interactions. Nevertheless, pressure of work meant that there were occasions when a considerable period of time lapsed between observation of the data and their recording.

All data was recorded manually, using a notepad. Sometimes the recording of data had to wait until the end of the day. Indeed, I rarely wrote up fieldnotes contemporaneously with the interactions I was recording. My fear was that constant, conspicuous note-taking of people's interactions would generate a perception of me as spy, rather than as research oriented professional (see Hunt 1984, and Brewer 1993 on the problems of the fieldworker being perceived as spy). Given such time lapses, it has to be conceded that some of the recordings were not verbatim, having been filtered through several hours of my memory (or lack of it) prior to their recording.

In common with much ethnography, most of my fieldnotes consisted of recordings of talk (Van Maanen 1981), although contextual descriptions were also included.

One of the disadvantages of locating my research in an ICU was that intensive care is in many ways unique as a therapeutic regime. As a consequence, considerable caution needs to be exercised in the extrapolation of results obtained from this specific situation to more general claims about the nature of nurse-doctor interactions. Three specificities pertinent to intensive care should be noted. First, the high level of medical intervention that intensive care entails means that there is far more interaction between nurses and doctors in an ICU than in most other types of unit, where a large proportion of care tends to be performed by nurses on their own. Second, emphasis on technology reinforces instrumental aspects of care, a factor which might be seen as strengthening medical superordination. Finally, the unit studied was fairly small, which meant that the number of personnel was rather low (39 nurses and 24 doctors). The smallness of this sample became especially problematic when examining sub-groups (for example, I only worked with three male nurses and five black doctors).

The grades of nurse working on the unit were: Nursing Sister, Staff Nurse, and Nursing Auxiliary. The grades of doctor were Consultant, Registrar, Senior House Officer. Because of the complexity and responsibility that intensive care was deemed to entail, Junior House Officers were not employed in the unit. For similar reasons, no Enrolled Nurses worked on the unit during my stay, although I am unsure whether this was because of a formal policy.

Informal interviews

As I have already noted, intensive care units are in many ways unique, leading to difficulties in the generalisation of conclusions from data drawn from them. It was clear that such data on their own, while interesting, would not be sufficient to ground the arguments that I wished to present. In order to overcome this problem, alternative sources of data were developed, most notably through the method of ethnographic interviewing. Thus, the specificity of the intensive care unit was compensated for by the diversity of the backgrounds of the nurses whom I interviewed.

The interviewees for ,my research consisted of 28 nurses from three units in a suburban general hospital (henceforth termed Suburban Hospital), which I interviewed in late 1992 and early 1993. All of these nurses were female. The grades interviewed were Enrolled Nurse, Staff Nurse, and Nursing Sister (Unit Co-Ordinator in the Nursing Development Unit). The units that the nurses worked on were:

1   A surgical ward, which dealt with general surgical cases which required more than one day admission.

2   A medical ward, which specialised in coronary care and which had a four-bedded coronary care unit, which was not officially recognised by the Health and Social Services Board as such (and therefore not funded to the level that an accredited coronary care unit would be).

3   A nursing development unit, which specialised in the rehabilitation of elderly patients, following treatment for acute conditions in other units.

All of these interviews were conducted on an informal basis, using an audio tape recorder. The topics covered ranged over a very broad area. I made no attempt to prevent nurses from discussing issues which they felt were pertinent to their occupational situation and their relationship with doctors or patients. Nor did I attempt to hide the specific aspects of interaction that I was interested in.

Permission to conduct the interviews was given by the hospital management on the understanding that each nurse should have the freedom to withhold consent to giving an interview. In line with this stricture, it was made clear to all that their participation was entirely voluntary. All the nurses I asked to talk to me consented to do so. However, I do not wish to give the impression that gaining acceptance from organisational gatekeepers exhausted the issue of access. As Johnson (1975) notes, trust is not a 'one-shot agreement'. At the start of each interview, I informed the person I was interviewing that their participation was confidential, and that while the information they gave me might be used in publications, their anonymity would be preserved, in that I would only use staff grading and sex to identify participants. I emphasised that neither doctors nor hospital management would have access to the transcripts of interviews. I believe that my explanations were successful in convincing nurses that I was not a spy in the camp (*cf.* Hunt 1984; Brewer 1993), and that as a consequence most were confident in talking to me.

The interviews took place on the wards in which the nurses worked, during their working hours. Most interviews took place either in nursing offices or staff rest rooms. At times this proved inconvenient for me in that interviews were often interrupted by my interviewees being called upon to perform clinical or administrative tasks. However, the converse of this was that my respondents were not greatly inconvenienced by my demands upon them.

College of Nursing

As part of a study of the socialisation of psychiatric nurses, I spent some time in 1990 and 1991 as a participant observer in a college of nursing which trained psychiatric nurses. I refer to the data gathered in this setting in Chapter Five to demonstrate the manner in which the occupational ethos of nursing is portrayed to students by nurse tutors. As this is the only use that I make of these data, I will gloss rapidly over the mechanics of the research. Briefly, I was allowed to sit in on classes over an extended period of time, openly recording what occurred. I was also able to interact informally with both staff and students during breaks. I found few problems in being accepted by students, although some of the teaching staff were wary of my recording them in teaching sessions. All participants concerned gave their consent to my being present.

Analysis

In line with the strictures of critical realism, I did not use the sort of inductivist method of analysis often associated with ethnography (Hammersley 1990). Rather, the process of analysis started with the production of synthetic *a priori* hypotheses about the nature of structures that would be likely to pertain in the social situation being examined. These hypotheses were subsequently tested through empirical examination of their effects.

The basic hypotheses I worked with were as follows:

1 Men are located in a structurally privileged social position in their relation to women.

2 Whites are located in a structurally privileged social position in their relation to blacks.

27

3   Relations of production pertaining in a given society will have an influence on
    the occupational position of welfare state employees.

From these hypotheses were developed lower-order hypotheses which will be discussed in the pertinent chapters.

From this point on, my method of analysis was more conventional, involving cycles of empirical testing and hypothetical reformulation. The process was, of course, not as mechanical as this; serendipity and imagination played a considerable part in the work's evolution. The cycle of testing and refining continued to the point of 'theoretical saturation' (Strauss 1987). However, while 'deviant' cases were examined to ascertain if they could be the basis of alternative explanations, my acceptance that social interaction takes place in an open system meant that I did not feel obliged to identify constant conjunctions in order to demonstrate the influence of social structures upon human agency.

My use of the empirical data that I had gathered was eclectic. Throughout the book, I shift from using transcripts of my participant observation fieldnotes to transcripts of interviews. My decisions about which to use rested simply on my evaluation of which pieces of data illustrated best the point that I was trying to make.

Personal reflexivity

A central aspect of reflexive accounts, that has been identified primarily by feminist researchers, is the uncovering of the person of the researcher. Williams (1993) notes that:

> 'the means of doing research' must include researchers' selves and experiences. From this perspective, primacy of experience can be read as a determination to practice personal reflexivity; that is to be aware of the ways in which self affects both research processes and outcomes, and to rigorously convey to readers of research accounts how this happens (1993:578).

It is to personal reflexivity that I now wish to turn. One of the most significant experiences pertaining to how I articulated with my field of study was the eight years that I spent as a clinical nurse, three years as a student nurse in England and five years as a staff nurse in the Suburban Hospital in which the interviews were conducted. This experience had a number of significant effects.

Occupational identity

First, my career as a nurse provided me with an occupational identity which, despite leaving the clinical field and entering the discipline of sociology, I have not lost. As a consequence, my perspective on the position of nursing and its relation to medicine is not a neutral one. As will become clear, my sentiments lie very much with nursing.

Given the power differential between doctors and nurses in favour of the former, I make no apology for my partisan position. I would concur with Becker that 'the question is not whether we should take sides, since we inevitably will, but rather whose side are we on' (1967:239). Given my continued occupational identity, my relationship with nursing is an 'organic' one, to use Gramsci's phrase.[5]

The direction of my sentiments, along with the continued effects of my former position as staff nurse had practical consequences upon the research, most notably in connection with my relationships with doctors. My initial plan was to interview both nurses and doctors in the Suburban Hospital about their perceptions of the relationship between the two occupations. However, after only three interviews with consultants that I had formerly worked with, it became very clear that this line of enquiry would produce very sparse results. To them, I remained a staff nurse who had gone off 'to do a course'. That I should be asking questions about how they articulated with nurses was seen as an impertinence. My attempts to bolster my status by managing my 'front' (Douglas 1972), using sharp suits, combed hair, university accreditation and the like, were to no avail. I was still seen (and very quickly began to see myself) as a nurse with ideas above his station. Moreover, the ethnographic approach that I was taking was seen by at least one consultant as scientifically invalid, and therefore not deserving of recognition.

After three unsatisfactory interviews, I decided to abandon this line of enquiry. I did so for three interrelated reasons. First, because I found the experience of the interviews personally uncomfortable. Second, I realised that, beyond confirming the existence of medical arrogance, they would yield little information of use. Third, and most importantly, I decided that I wished to concentrate my examination of the position of nursing from the perspective of nurses.

A more positive result of my nursing experience was the fact that I remained (and continue to be) registered on Part 2 of the United Kingdom Central Council for Nursing, Midwifery and Health Visiting's professional register. This meant that I could enter the field as a participant. Moreover, my nursing experience meant that I required little time to familiarise myself with the social situation that I was examining.

Native ethnography?

Another effect of my experience as a nurse was that it gave me an insider's perspective of the occupational field that I was studying. This meant that the boundary between myself as a researcher and those being researched was blurred.[6] This is not to say that I have written an ethnography unproblematically from a native's point of view. Even during participant observation, when I was practising as a nurse, I remained also a sociologist and ethnographer, holding the perspectives associated with such a position. This particular position as ethnographer returning to a field within which I was once a native was not without its tensions (*cf.* Williams 1990). At different times, one or other of the roles were dominant. Being in the field

29

as participant observer in the Metropolitan Hospital for an extended period of time had the effect of reinforcing my native identity. As time went on, it became more and more difficult for me to maintain my sociological imagination. I experienced an increasing tendency to take aspects of my social situation for granted. Elements that, on entering the field I would have found noteworthy, I began to see as 'natural'. This was indicated by a steady decrease in the volume of my fieldnotes, which it took more and more discipline to complete.

Conversely, being out of the field, working within a sociological milieu, reinforced my detachment from nursing. Whether or not this detachment during the period of 'writing up' led to an unwarranted cynicism in places, I will leave the reader to judge.

Power and research

I noted above that my attempts to use front management techniques such as power dressing to reinforce my independent status as sociologist to consultants met with little success. Foolishly, I initially attempted to try the same trick with the Suburban Hospital nurses that I wished to interview. Fortunately, it was as unsuccessful with them as it was with the doctors. On entering one ward in formal dress, I encountered a former colleague, whom I had not seen for five years. Without a word, she came up to me, took hold of both my trouser legs at the knee, hoisted my trousers up, and exclaimed:

Transcript 2\1
Nursing Development Unit

SN(F)   Jesus Christ, he hasn't even got odd socks on. By Christ, boy, you really think you're something now.

Moments after, another former colleague who worked as a domestic assistant on the unit came round the corner with a tea trolley. Her response was equally unimpressed:

Transcript 2\2
Nursing Development Unit

D(F)   Will you look at the shape of him, with his snazzy suit. You'd hardly think that he used to be the NUPE Branch Secretary. Another bloody traitor off to management. You're all the same, you men. Off and away up the ladder and leave us poor sods to do the work.

SP   No, no, I'm not in management. I'm working in the University.

D(F)   Same difference. I'm still pushing the tea trolley. Yous are all the same, yous men.

I should point out that this interaction was not nearly as aggressive as it reads. Nevertheless, it highlights a number important issues. First, there was little evidence that my rapport with people in the field was compromised by their perception of a power differential between us. As far as they were concerned, my 'master status' (Hughes 1945) remained largely as it had been during the period in which I was an employee of the hospital.

Second, it indicates that Warren and Rasmussen's contention that 'matters of dress, demeanour, and conversational style [of the researcher] can be altered to fit the setting' (1977:350) was not appropriate to my situation. Many of the nurses interviewed already had a fixed conception of my 'natural' demeanour. My attempts to alter this were quickly seen as disingenuous. Despite my initial *faux pas*, this was a major boon to my research, in that both myself and my respondents saw the interviews as unstrained conversations between former colleagues.

The male researcher

The above transcript also indicates the importance of another aspect of myself, namely my maleness, which differentiated me from the vast majority of people that I was researching. Nursing is an occupation numerically dominated by women. As such it is unfavourably located within the social structure of patriarchy. Men enjoy positions of dominance over female nurses both within the occupation and from without, (see Chapter Six for a fuller discussion of this issue). As someone who had moved from clinical nursing into academia, I was viewed by at least one nurse as benefiting from my privileged gendered position.

Transcript 2\3
Medical Ward

SN(F)   Are you glad to be out of nursing?

SP   Well, to be honest, there are some things I really miss. The interaction with people. But there are certainly things I don't. Getting in here for half seven in the morning and not getting away until nine. I'm getting too long in the tooth for that sort of thing.

SN(F)   Hmmm, I don't want to be sexist, but that's what a lot of male nurses do, isn't it - get out to education.

Given that I was perceived by some nurses as benefiting from my masculinity, it is incumbent upon me to ask whether or not, as a man, I am in a position to comment upon the experiences of women.[7] There is certainly a strain of thought within nursing feminist writers which would argue that I am not. Thus Webb notes that 'the overwhelming majority of [feminist] writers ... take the view that men cannot take part in feminist research as researchers' (1993:417). The dangers become all the more acute when it is considered that men dominate nursing academic discourse out of all proportion to their numbers as practitioners (Ryan and Porter 1993; Porter 1995).

My response to this challenge is tentative. I do not wish to deny that the sex of the 'knower' is of considerable significance. However, while it is important, I do not believe that it has an absolutely deterministic effect. As Code argues:

> Understanding the circumstances of the knower makes possible a more *discerning* evaluation. The claim that certain of those circumstances are epistemologically significant - the sex of the knower in this instance - by no means implies that they are definitive, capable of bearing the entire burden of justification and evaluation ... But claiming that the circumstances of the knower are not epistemologically definitive is quite different from claiming that they are of no epistemological consequence ... [T]he sex of the knower is one of a cluster of *subjective* factors ... constitutive of received conceptions of knowledge and of what it means to be a knower (1991:4, emphasis in original).

Given the importance of the subjective factor of my gender, how do I justify my presumption to write about, and try to explain, the experiences of female nurses? One possible route is to follow Connell (1989), who argues that while men are advantaged by the social structures that currently pertain, and therefore have a broad interest in maintaining the *status quo*, there are other circumstances in men's biographies that may militate towards an interest in change.

In relation to the specific social situation being examined here, it might be noted that while male nurses *qua* men have different interests to their female colleagues, *qua* nurses they have much in common. However, even if we accept this line of argument, there remains a gap centred around differing gender interests.

A stronger line returns to the Enlightenment project of human emancipation. This project has been forcefully reiterated by Doyal and Gough (1991) through their theory of human need. Doyal and Gough demur at the validity of what they term 'group relativism', that is entailed in the assumption that 'women's experiences constitute a different view of reality, an entirely different ontology or way of going about making sense of the world' (Stanley and Wise 1983:117). Doyal and Gough argue that the assertion of moral autonomy by groups such as women is politically counter-productive, in that it leads to the inability of members of one group to justifiably criticise the activities of any other.

This moral incommensurability comes into stark focus when a clash occurs between the values of different oppressed groups. Thus, for example, for feminists to take a relativist position means that they have no grounds upon which to criticise practices such as purdah or female circumcision, for in doing so they leave themselves open to charges of ethnocentrism by relativist anti-racists. Criticism of such practices, then, must rest on an assertion that they are objectively oppressive and harmful, irrespective of which cultural group engages in them.

This leads Doyal and Gough to the conclusion that, while they may be articulated in culturally different ways, all human beings have basic objective needs. They classify these needs under the headings of physical health and autonomy. Thus, the criterion for judging social research moves from (literally) *ad hominem* arguments, to assessment on the basis of the position researchers take *vis-a-vis* the promotion of objective human needs.

'Race' and class

Mutatis mutandis, the same defence can be used in relation to other aspects of my biography that entail a privileged social position. Thus, despite arguments by some anti-racists on the ineffability of black culture to whites (for example, Shah 1989), I presume to tackle the issue of racism in nurse-doctor relations. I do so not on the basis of some arrogant claim that I am able to gain an absolute phenomenological understanding of Black experience; clearly I cannot (Cashmore 1982). My more modest task is to elucidate the nature of interactions between whites and blacks.

Similarly, as someone in an economically cosseted position, I address the topic of class relations. Here, I think the gap between my experience and that of my respondents was narrowest. Certainly, the more senior clinical nursing staff were on a higher wage than the one I enjoy. In addition, as I have already noted, staff's perception of my status was largely generated from their experience of working with me as a colleague, rather than their interactions with me as a university lecturer.

Critical realism and human emancipation

To return to the project of critical realism, despite the differences in my social position to that of the people I was interviewing, my justification for conducting this research is that by exposing the structural relationships that are constraining the members of the social groups that I am studying, I am making a small contribution towards the possibility of their resolution. Bhaskar (1989a) argues that to be free is to know, to possess the opportunity, and to be disposed to act in one's real interests. This book may provide nurses with more knowledge about their situation, may help them to identify the opportunities and restraints that their social position entails, and may even persuade some to be disposed to change.

In conclusion, I reiterate that my justificatory argument is a tentative one. Notwithstanding the aforementioned philosophical defence of my position, I have no wish to deny that the social statuses ascribed to me within society had an effect upon my interactions with others. They most certainly did. However, I hope that, by providing a biographical outline, I have 'made possible a more discerning evaluation' (Code 1991:4) by the reader. It is for the reader to decide whether or not my specific position within the social structure has led to distortions in my analysis.

Notes

1. Hammersley is not, of course, the only ethnographic critic of ethnography. Other notable examples include Atkinson (1990) and Woolgar (1988).

2. The idea that we identify laws through the perception of constant conjunctions comes from David Hume. He explains his argument thus:

> We remember to have had frequent instances of the existence of one species of objects; and also remember, that the individuals of another species of objects have always attended them, and have existed in a regular order of contiguity and succession with regard to them ... [W]e call one the *cause* and the other *effect*, and infer the existence of the one from that of the other ... Thus in advancing we have insensibly discovered a new relation betwixt cause and effect ... This relation is their CONSTANT CONJUNCTION. Contiguity and succession are not sufficient to make us pronounce any two objects to be cause and effect, unless we perceive, that these two relations are preserv'd in several instances (1969: 135-6, emphasis in original).

3. By reverse archaeology, I understand Stanley to mean that the biographer should attempt to build up the complexity of the lives of the people they write about, rather than analysing them down to what she would see as unwarranted and simplistic essentials.

4. Bhaskar qualifies his argument about the necessity of knowledge for emancipation by noting that knowledge is not sufficient. He argues that 'to be free is (i) to know, (ii) to possess the opportunity and (iii) to be disposed to act in (or towards) one's real interests (1989a: 89-90).

5. Gramsci explains his concept of the organic intellectual as follows:

> Every social group, coming into existence on the original terrain of an essential function in the world of economic production, creates together with itself, organically, one or more strata of intellectuals which give it homogeneity and an awareness of its own function not only in the economic but also in the social and political fields (1971:5).

   Perhaps I flatter myself.

6. In terms of Gold's (1958) typology, my role lay somewhere between 'complete participant', in that I was a fully-fledged member of the group under study, and 'participant-as-observer', in that those that I was studying were aware that ours was a fieldwork relationship.

7. Problems, of course, are encountered by female researchers attempting to examine predominantly male cultures (cf. Hunt 1984). However, because of the power differentials resulting from patriarchy, this issue is qualitatively different.

Part Two
THE DEVELOPMENT OF NURSE-DOCTOR RELATIONS

3 A historical review

Introduction

The aim of this chapter is to examine the historical relationship between doctors and nurses. This will be done by reviewing the appropriate literature. Most attention will be paid to the immediate past quarter of a century, although there will be a brief review of literature pertaining to an earlier era. For analysis of the recent period, I have chosen 1967 as the historical base line because it was in that year that Leonard Stein published his seminal paper on the 'doctor-nurse game'. The contention of my argument about the nature of nurse-doctor relations will be, firstly, that it has been changing over time, and secondly, that the direction of that change has been towards a more egalitarian form of communication.

I should admit from the start that at times the reader may find my empirical evidence rather scanty. This is an unfortunate inevitability, because, as Hughes (1988) has noted, the nature of everyday nurse-doctor interactions has received surprisingly little attention in the literature.

The doctor-nurse game

Stein (1978 [1967]) argued that interactions between nurses and doctors were governed by the rules of an intricate game. The reasons for, and nature of the doctor-nurse game are given by him as follows.

While doctors have total responsibility for making decisions about the care of patients, they require comprehensive data on which to base their decisions. These data are obtained from a number of sources, including recommendations from nurses. Yet, the idea of a nurse openly recommending a course of action to a physician is almost too outrageous to contemplate. Such assertiveness would contravene the tenets that both groups of workers have been socialised into during their occupational training.

On entering college, medical students soon learn that their prospective occupation involves risks with very high stakes for their clients. A medical mistake can be a matter of life and death. The death of a patient is a traumatic event for a physician - as Stein colourfully puts it, 'when a child dies, some of him dies too' (1978:112). As a result, the burden of the possibility of a mistake can become unbearable. The way in which doctors tend to cope with their fear of failure is to avoid it by cultivating the pretence of omnipotence and omniscience. This pretence of absolute knowledge and power can only work if those around doctors play along with it. Hence the significance of nurses' subservience. If a nurse voiced an open recommendation, the medical posture of omniscience would be threatened.

Conversely, nurses' training involves the inculcation of military style discipline and a reverential attitude to medical colleagues. As one of Stein's interviewees put it, 'He's God Almighty and your job is to wait on him' (1978:115). So, just as medical students are taught to regard the idea of an open suggestion from a non-physician as an inexcusable effrontery, nurses would be equally horrified by the prospect, believing that it would be tantamount to suggesting that their betters did not know their business.

The problem with this kind of absolute dominance and subordination is that it sits ill with the pragmatic requirements of doctors' and nurses' work. For doctors, avoiding the fear of failure through the pretence of omnipotence is not enough. They also have to make sure that they do not fail too often in reality. They therefore strive to give the best care they are capable of. To do this, they need to be open to input from the people who are with patients most, namely nurses. Similarly, nurses are imbued with a strong sense of responsibility for the well-being of patients, a responsibility that they discharge by assisting the physician in his treatment.

Thus, members of both occupations are caught in a paradox. On the one hand, the doctor is supposed to be omniscient. On the other hand, the nurse is supposed to be able, and indeed required, to make a significant contribution to care.

According to Stein, this paradox is resolved by means of playing the doctor-nurse game, the object of which is to allow nurses to make significant recommendations to their medical colleagues, while at the same time appearing passive. The rules of the game are clear:

> The cardinal rule of the game is that open disagreement between the players must be avoided at all costs. Thus, the nurse can communicate her recommendations without appearing to make a recommendation statement. The physician, in requesting a recommendation from a nurse, must do so without appearing to be asking for it (1978:110).

This is usually achieved by nurses substituting statements about patients' conditions which implicitly carry a recommendation for more direct forms of speech. This allows physicians to co-opt the implied recommendation and voice it as their own.

The historical location of the doctor-nurse game

Before going on to discuss how the literature has interpreted the nature of nurse-doctor interactions since the publication of Stein's paper, it is interesting to speculate on whether or not the game was a phenomenon that emerged during the era in which Stein was writing, or whether it was a long-established convention. Unfortunately, the data that can be called upon to illuminate this question is rather thin. There is, however, at least one study which examines the nurse-doctor relationship from an historical perspective (Keddy *et al.* 1986). This study was based on interviews with Canadian nurses who had worked or trained during the 1920s and 1930s. Keddy *et al.* are quite explicit about the form of occupational relations in that era: 'In analysing the data, it becomes apparent that most of the nurses interviewed were involved in the interactive methods of the doctor-nurse game' (1986: 748).

On face value, it would seem that Stein has identified a relatively immutable phenomenon. However, close examination of Keddy *et al.*'s evidence suggests that the game was not in fact being played; that nurses in this era did not even have the opportunity to indulge in the making of covert recommendations.

Keddy *et al.* demonstrate that three of the rules of the game were adhered to, namely that nurses were expected to show doctors respect, that they could not openly diagnose or make recommendations to doctors, and that open disagreement or confrontation was forbidden. These rules all related to one side of the paradox that the doctor-nurse game is purported to resolve; they all have the effect of reinforcing physicians' sense of omnipotence. However, Keddy *et al.* supply little empirical evidence that the other side of the paradox, that 'The nurse is to be bold, have initiative, and be responsible for making significant recommendations' (Stein 1978:109) was accommodated in nurse-physician relations, as recounted by their interviewees. Indeed the two examples they give relating to position of nurses in decision making processes would seem to indicate that nurses' contribution was negligible. The first example demonstrates that while the nurses might have had recommendations that they wished to make, they had no opportunity to do so even by covert means.

> Nurses have always had ideas and improvements in mind, based on what they knew and saw in the clinical setting. A nurse referred to two different methods of treating pneumonia that she used in the same ward, depending on which doctor the patient had. 'Dr Jones' [patients] got along a lot better with their treatment of fresh air ... or I felt they did.' With what we know today about treating pneumonia, her observation and ensuing opinion is substantiated. Unfortunately in her time, nurses did not voice their opinions. While she was aware of the most effective treatment she would not have dared to discuss it with the other physicians (1986:749).

Given that the nurse continued to operate a regime that she disagreed with, we can conclude that not only was she unable to effect change by direct intervention, she was equally unable to utilise the subtleties of the doctor-nurse game to change treatment.

The second example given by Keddy *et al.* indicates that the only way that nurses could implement actions which they thought were proper, was not to recommend their use by playing the doctor-nurse game, but to simply go behind the doctors' backs and carry out the actions secretly.

> One nurse said that although a particular physician did not want his pneumonia patients bathed for long periods of time she would nonetheless give them daily baths. Upon being asked what the physician said about that, she said she would not tell him. She said 'Well, the doctor didn't know it - it was done when he wasn't there' (1986:750).

The powerlessness experienced by nurses in this period suggests that the use of the doctor-nurse game, while it still embodies extreme inequality, is actually indicative of a degree of democratisation in the nurse-doctor relationship. At least it entails the possibility of participation by means of covert recommendation, rather than total exclusion from decision making.

The impression of almost total subservience is reinforced by Darbyshire, who cites extracts from turn-of-the-century American medical journals. For example:

> Every attempt at initiative on the part of the nurse should be reproved by the physicians. [1901]

> The instinct of the eternal feminine for sacrificial service has been [the nurse's] sole saving grace ... no calling may more fitly adopt the noble motto of the noblest line of the kingly servants of man 'I serve' [1913] (1987:32).

The second extract above indicates that one of the crucial determining factors in nurses' subservience was the extreme repressiveness of gender roles during this era. Doctors were able to make very effective use of gender stereotypes to justify the power that they wielded. It should be noted that their formal power was considerable. For example, the doctors in Keddy *et al.*'s study had control both over the education of nurses and their hiring and firing.

However, even in the early part of this century, there were signs that nurses were not prepared to be as subservient as doctors might have wished. From a base-line of almost total subordination, nurses were beginning to shift the rules of engagement in their favour. One of the first changes in the etiquette of interaction recalled by Keddy *et al.*'s interviewees was that nurses ceased to stand up in the presence of doctors. This piece of symbolic rebellion caused puzzlement and consternation, as one nurse recalled.

> The medical staff in the beginning didn't understand what we were doing. They were still used to nurses standing up when they came to the desk. This was stopped and they didn't like that (1986:751).

This sort of informal, particular rebellion was founded upon more generalised moves on the part of nursing entrepreneurs to improve the status of their occupation. In America, this struggle was largely concentrated around the issue of 'professional' education, with the first collegiate school of nursing being founded in the University of Minnesota as early as 1909 (Jensen 1959). In Britain, most energy was expended on the attainment of a 'professional' register (cf. Baly 1980; Witz 1992). While the emphasis may have been on different strategies, it is clear that on both sides of the Atlantic, the aspiration of nurses to narrow the gap between themselves and their medical colleagues has been long-standing.

Gradual change

While I cannot claim that the evidence that I have presented here is conclusive, I would argue that there are strong indications that between the 1930s and the 1960s, nurse-doctor relations gradually shed some of their authoritarian characteristics. The doctor-nurse game can be seen as part of this process. It stands as an intermediate stage between the total absence of nursing rights to participate in decision making, and the right to openly voice recommendations.

The changing nature of relations

This section will examine how the dynamics of nurse-doctor relations have fared since 1967. In order to give some idea of development, I will somewhat arbitrarily divide the literature into two sub-sections - that published prior to 1980, and that published after.

The 1960s and 1970s

The first thing to note is that during this era, nurses began to develop a new strategy to attain occupational autonomy. This strategy emerged in North America. Reflecting this, literature about nurse-doctor relationships that was published during the 1960s and 1970s emanates almost exclusively from there. With educationalists in the vanguard, the aim of this strategy was to carve out for nursing a sphere of professional autonomy. The fundamental mechanism to achieve this aim was the nursing process, which, with its five steps of data collection, diagnosis, planning, treatment and evaluation, provided a systematic framework for nursing practice (Glanze *et al.* 1986). Upon the foundations of the process were built two interrelated strategies for the advancement of nursing, the whole package going under the epithet of 'New Nursing' (Salvage 1992).

The first strategy might be described as the accumulation of intellectual capital. This entailed both the commandeering of insights from disciplines outside nursing, such as sociology and psychology, in order to develop a knowledge base for nursing (cf. Perry and Jolley 1991), and the development of nursing theory, most notably through the construction of models for nursing practice (cf. Kershaw and Salvage 1986). Predicated upon the expansion of knowledge were demands for more academically orientated training for nurses, which led eventually in Britain to the adoption of the Project 2000 educational reforms.

The second strategy involved the development of an ideology of partnership between nurses and patients, whereby patients were encouraged to actively participate in their care, rather than be the passive recipients of medical-style paternalism (Salvage 1992).

Chapter Four will include a fuller discussion of these developments. For the moment, I will largely confine discussion to the nursing process itself.

The nursing process

The significance of the nursing process lies in its claim that diagnosis and subsequent prescription is a nursing prerogative. This claim to a diagnostic role for nurses goes to the heart of medical dominance, because one of the fundamental bases of that dominance is doctors' control over diagnosis. For any health problem, action stems from diagnosis, and because of this the diagnostician will assume an authoritative role in his/her relationships with both clients and allied occupations (Terence Johnson 1972).

The process was first mooted in the American literature in a paper by Lydia Hall as early as 1955 (Iyer *et al.* 1986). However, it took a long time to develop from the purely conceptual to the practical. It was not until the 1970s that it began to make an significant impact in clinical settings. While the academic literature on the process grew considerably during the 1960s, and while that literature was increasingly taught to students, the process remained primarily a teaching tool, rarely being used to organise care on hospital wards (de la Cuesta 1983). The occupational entrepreneurs who were promoting the nursing process hailed overwhelmingly from the educational sector. That said, it was highly unlikely to have succeeded as it did in becoming part of official clinical philosophy, had it not been seen as beneficial by managerial elites. When it finally arrived on the wards, as well as organising care, it was used as a managerial tool to itemise, monitor and cost nursing services (Dingwall *et al.* 1988). It is hardly a coincidence that it began to enjoy an increasingly hegemonic position in service institutions in the mid-1970s, a period when the fiscal crises of Western states led to concerns about the escalating costs of health care (cf. O'Connor 1976).

In 1973, the proponents of the process gained a significant victory when the American Nurses' Association adopted the process in its *Standards of Nursing Practice* (Kenney 1991). Ubiquitous adoption of the nursing process in American Nursing was ensured shortly after, when the Commission responsible for the licensing of hospitals made the preparation of care plans a prerequisite for the accreditation of nursing services (de la Cuesta 1983).

The idea of the nursing process was not taken up in Britain until 20 years after Hall's initial formulation in 1955. However, while interest in it was late to develop, once it became part of nursing discourse, its practical adoption followed with spectacular swiftness. The first articles on the process were not published in British journals until 1975. By 1977, it was being introduced into clinical areas, and was included in the general nurse training syllabus (de la Cuesta 1983). By 1983, under the terms of the Nurses, Midwives and Health Visitors Act, it had become a legally prescribed activity.[1]

Power on the wards

The question of importance here is whether the occupational projects of nursing educationalists and academics actually delivered the goods for clinical nurses who were involved in day-to-day interactions with doctors. Certainly, as far as the early stages are concerned, examination of the literature leads to the conclusion that they did not. In her description of the institutional position of nurses in the USA, Devine noted that:

> Nursing educators have developed the ideology of the 'professional' nurses with indispensable knowledge, demanding autonomous decision-making authority. Staff nurses in the organization, however, are often confronted with their own powerlessness with regard to policy-making, implementing change with regard to rules and regulations, or even which of their skills can be utilized in the hospital setting. The result is confusion with the ambiguity that exists between ideology and structure (1978:289).

The dichotomy between ideological aspirations and material reality identified by Devine left clinical nurses in an impossible dilemma. It may be that, in order to avoid the consequences of this dilemma, many nurses were less than enthusiastic about the aspirations of nursing entrepreneurs.

> Collaboration between the professions [of nursing and medicine] and collegial relationships between its members are advanced by innovative, idealistic educators, administrators, and organizers in nursing. But there are precious few supporters of this line of thinking in medicine or, indeed, among the rank and file of nurses (Hoekelman 1975:1150).

That many nurses were unenthusiastic about promoting more equal inter-professional relationships should not necessarily be taken as an indication that, given the opportunity, they would not have wanted more equality. As Devine (1978) argued, the structural reality of the institutions that most nurses worked in was such that there was simply no possibility of them being able to treat doctors (or be treated by them) as collegial equals. It could well have been the case that many nurses, realising that this sort of relationship was out of their grasp, felt uncomfortable with the cognitive dissonance that resulted from the discrepancy between an attitude of equality and unequal behaviour. Because they could do little about the behaviour,

43

the only way they could reduce dissonance was by altering their attitudes (cf. Festinger 1957).[2]

The discomfort that falling between the stools of educators' aspirations and doctors' expectations was illustrated by Logan in her description of the experience of the new nursing graduate on her arrival in the clinical arena

> who thinks of herself as a novice on the health team but with an equal and unique contribution to make as a nurse. Immediately, the novice practitioner must work with a physician who has a very traditional frame of reference regarding the nurse. The new graduate is quickly aware of how much she needs the doctor in an acute care situation but she does not know the rules involved in keeping this relationship functioning smoothly. This fact was clear during a recent orientation program this writer attended. Three-quarters of a group of ... graduates had had a confrontation with a physician before the three-week orientation was finished (1976:5).

Given this level of friction with members of a more powerful occupational group, it is hardly surprising that nurses began to back away from their aspirations for equality of relationships with doctors. Indeed, Logan herself epitomises this type of sour grape retrenchment. Her answer to the dilemma was that, because nurses could not get away with rejecting their role as doctors' handmaidens, the only thing for it was to make sure that they were properly trained to carry out the servile roles expected of them, at least until doctors could be persuaded that nurses deserved better: 'Considering that nurses need physicians, ... nursing educators must retain handmaiden skills in the curriculum until they are not so urgently required' (1976:25).

This is not to say that all nurses were cowed by medical disapproval of their audacity. There were a number of attempts in specific institutions to carve out new, more egalitarian forms of interaction (Lewis *et al.* 1969; Mauksch and Young 1974; Thomstad *et al.* 1975). Nevertheless, these were self-conscious, isolated efforts which had little immediate effect in changing the general culture of nurse-doctor relationships.

Despite the attempts of nursing entrepreneurs to gain recognition for overt nursing involvement in decisions about patient care, the reality for many nurses, even in America, remained stuck in the doctor-nurse game. A number of commentators explicitly identify the game as the most prevalent mode of interaction, for example:

> [Medical] cooperation is often only obtained by playing the 'doctor-nurse game' (Hoekelman 1975:1150).

> Another result of nurse passivity and physician dominance is what has been called the doctor-nurse game (Kalisch and Kalisch 1982a [1977]).

It should not, however, be thought that nursing was trapped in a limbo, unable to progress beyond *sub rosa* involvement in decision making. The very fact that Stein and other commentators were addressing the issue was in itself progress.

Most of these commentaries were quite explicit in their evaluation of the manner in which most nurses interacted with their medical colleagues. Stein himself described the game as a 'transactional neurosis', and argued that 'both professions would enhance themselves by taking steps to change the attitudes which breed the game' (1978:117). Kalisch and Kalisch were even more withering in their attack upon sexist assumptions about the natural basis of nurses' deference to doctors:

> [W]e have somehow discovered that nurses, who are still overwhelmingly women, do not faint from the strain of analytical thinking or necessarily lose the 'delicate bloom of womanhood' in the process, and that the questioning of incongruous professional relationships will not yield a drastic decline in the marriage rate and promote 'race suicide' (1982a:221).

We might summarise the position during the 1970s as being one where American nurses at least were becoming increasingly aware of, and frustrated by, medical expectations that they should act in a subservient manner. Not only were many openly complaining about this state of affairs; some were also trying to implement formal, practical procedures which would allow nurses to close the power gap and to create some autonomous space to work within. However, efforts to promote change were severely hampered by social and institutional structures which militated in support of continuing medical dominance.

1980 to the present

In the early 1980s, the debate about the relative occupational positions of doctors and nurses, most notably as a consequence of the nursing process, began to become something of an issue in British nursing and medical literature. The nursing process was first introduced to clinical settings in 1977, and by the early 1980s its formal adoption was approaching universality. It was at this point that its importance vis-à-vis nurse-doctor relations began to sink in.

Interpreting the process

During the first half of the 1980s, the issue of the nursing process became the battle ground on which the contest for power between nurses and doctors was played.

On the one hand, some nursing writers attempted to rally their colleagues around the process as a weapon to free themselves from blind obedience to their medical colleagues (for example, Iveson-Iveson 1981). It was argued that adoption of the nursing process 'would give nurses autonomy and to a considerable extent remove medical constraints' (Bowman 1983:10). Extolling of the virtues of the process was often accompanied by exposure of the weaknesses of medicine (for example, Boylan

45

1982). Few of the sacred cows of medicine were left untainted. Even doctors' role as hospital gatekeepers was seen as up for grabs:

> The fact that patients are admitted to hospital, generally by a doctor, does not give them [doctors] any rights or control over the patient. It is purely the bureaucratic process that exists for gaining access to our health care system ... What is wrong with a nurse deciding to admit a patient to hospital for nursing?' (Ride 1983:12).[3]

This sort of naive militancy may not have been the most politic tactic for nursing entrepreneurs to take. It served both to alert doctors to the threat that was being posed, and to alienate many of them from the nursing process.

One of the first indications of medical awareness of the possible ramifications of the nursing process was contained in an editorial in the *British Medical Journal* (BMJ) in 1981, which noted that doctors were largely unaware of the major changes occurring in nursing, and warned that these changes could have a profound effect upon nurse-doctor relations. The consequent correspondence to the BMJ was split between those who supported a move towards multidisciplinary health care, and those who wished to go back to the days when everybody knew their place (Clifford 1985). While it is not possible to calculate from the literature which point of view was in the ascendancy, from the expressions of dissatisfaction published in the medical press over the next few years (for example, Anonymous 1983; Mitchell 1984), we can conclude at the very least that the nursing process was not being met with universal sanguinity by doctors.

That this unease was shared by the senior echelons of the medical establishment was demonstrated when a confidential circular issued by the British Medical Association's Central Committee for Hospital Medical Services in 1983, which was critical of the nursing process, was leaked to the *Nursing Mirror* (Walton 1986).

In reading the nostalgic musings of doctors who yearned for a return to the position they once enjoyed (or were about to lose), we get a good impression both of just how much influence medicine once had over nursing, and how this influence was being attenuated over time:

> many of us have felt anxious for some time ...[about] the progressive exclusion of doctors from nursing affairs. In many hospitals (but not, I am glad to say, in my own) doctors have been removed from the appointment committees which choose ward sisters and nurse managers, and in many hospitals, including my own, have been virtually excluded from nurse teaching ... In my view the background and training of the nurse teachers does not allow them to act as substitutes for doctors in the teaching about diagnosis and outcome (Mitchell 1984:217).

This kind of pomposity was only one approach that medical detractors of the nursing project took. Another was patronising facetiousness:

And what does it [the nursing process] all mean to doctors? Most likely not much: most are probably unaware of it ... Those of my colleagues ... who took exception to it seemed to be responding not to the nursing process itself, which is essentially laudable and entirely unthreatening, but to a kind of militant tendency within nursing that has mistaken the nursing process for something bigger. This aberration ... sees in the nursing process something like liberation theology or a revolutionary philosophy. I don't think it's there, even if you look closely, but there are steely eyed nurses who think it is ... but let us hope ... that it's only a phase and they'll get through it (Currie, 1984:1219).

The vigorousness of medical opposition led some to believe that nurses had overplayed their hand: 'it seems, nurses could have done themselves ... more harm than good by over-emphasising the 'autonomous' aspect of the nursing process' (Walton 1986:11).

There were those within nursing who thought that a unilateral declaration of independence was not a feasible option. The extension of nursing autonomy depended on the assent of the hitherto dominant occupation in health care:

The transfer of authority, accountability, and responsibility to clinical nurses can only be achieved effectively if other disciplines, particularly medicine, both understand and accept this change (Royal College of Nursing Committee on Standards of Nursing Care 1981:10).

Increasingly, the rhetoric of nursing entrepreneurs emphasised the concept of teamwork, rather than the clarion call to nursing independence. This was the line taken by Tierney (1984) and Rowden (1984) in their replies to Mitchell:[4]

When there are shades of grey ... where no single profession can claim a monopoly over wisdom, openness and mutual trust between the professions will ensure that the patient gets the best that is available ... I can assure readers that relationships between nurses and doctors at the Royal Marsden [where the nursing process is in use] are sound, the best I have experienced; the nursing process does not have to threaten these relationships (Rowden 1984:220-221).

This emphasis on co-operation was taken up by sectors in both the medical and nursing establishment, with publications emanating from a joint conference on interaction between nurses and doctors (Duncan and McLachan 1984), and from the deliberations of the Nuffield Working Party on Communication (Walton and McLachan 1986). While accepting that friction existed, many of the eminent contributors were of the opinion that, given the right attitudes and sufficient mutual understanding, the relationship between nurses and doctors could be a successful one.

It was not only doctors who were questioning the nursing process. Even while its promulgators were hailing it as the road to freedom, other nurses were expressing doubts. Nursing objections, however, were made on different grounds to those given by doctors. The fundamental problem that nursing critics had was simply that the nursing process did not deliver what had been promised of it. Rather than acting as an effective tool for autonomous professional practice, it was seen by some as yet another unreflexive ritual, and little more than a paper exercise (cf. Gooch 1982; McFarlane 1983; Wilkinson 1983). By 1986, a major report commissioned by the Department of Health and Social Security came to the depressing conclusion that: 'As yet it is not possible to say with any conviction that implementation of the nursing process has improved the lot of the patients' (Hayward 1986:39).

Changes in day-to-day relationships

We have seen that at a macro-level, a number of conflicting currents were affecting the relationship between medicine and nursing. At least five camps have been identified, three in nursing and two in medicine. In nursing, there were those who enthusiastically promoted the nursing process as a weapon to independently empower nurses; there were those who promoted the process to empower nurses through the development of multidisciplinary decision making; and finally there were those who were unconvinced that the nursing process was workable. The medical side was divided between those who were prepared to allow nurses a greater degree of involvement in decision making, and those who wished to hold on to their traditional authority.

The aim of this section is to examine the literature which gives an indication of how nurses and doctors were interacting at a day-to-day level while these sectors competed for influence.

When nurse knows best

One of the few qualitative analyses of the character of everyday interactions between doctors and nurses was published by David Hughes in 1988. The empirical information it was based on, however, was gathered in the late 1970s. The aim of the paper was to describe the central feature of inter-occupational interaction in the casualty department of a British district general hospital.

Taking the frequent references in the literature to the doctor-nurse game as his starting point, Hughes argued that unqualified acceptance of Stein's thesis demonstrated an unwarranted assumption of homogeneity in the division of labour, which ignored the situated nature of the relationship between nurses and doctors. His own paper came to a different conclusion about the character of interactions:

> The present study portrays the nurse-doctor relationship in terms of a gradient of behaviour. Sometimes, in much the same way that Stein's (1967) account of

the 'doctor-nurse game' suggests, recommendations take the form of subtle cues or cryptic references to information unearthed by the nurse. But for much of the time nurses seem much less preoccupied with concealing their role as advice-givers than the 'game' metaphor suggests. Nurses, even while acknowledging the doctor's clinical authority, frequently offer advice on many aspects of departmental practice in an open and straightforward way. More rarely, senior nursing staff intervene quite bluntly to point out shortcomings in the work of certain junior doctors, and effectively take control of the processing of particular patients (1988:16-17).

The impact of a number of exigencies related to the particular setting that Hughes studied, meant that medical dominance was often attenuated in informal interactions. Primary among the exigencies identified by Hughes were the volume of clientele coming through the department, which meant that doctors had to rely on nurses to doing a considerable amount of informal triaging, in order to make their own workload manageable; the fact that the turnover of medical staff was far greater than that of nursing staff, which resulted in nurses being the repositories of departmental customs and practices; the fact that many of the doctors were either very junior, or were 'rusty' general practitioner locums, who therefore looked to nurses for guidance; and finally, the fact that many of the doctors were immigrants from the Indian sub-continent, who sometimes relied on nurses for cultural translation.

While Hughes's point about being wary of nomothetic extrapolations from the results of particular studies is an important one, I would argue that there are general lessons to be learnt from his paper. Its significance lies in that it was the exception that broke the rule. Hughes demonstrated that, given auspicious circumstances, nurses did not feel compelled to play the doctor-nurse game. While there may have been many hospital wards in the late 1970s where the game remained the prevalent mode of interaction, the fact that on some wards this was no longer the case in-dicated that medical dominance was being further weakened.

Plus ça change ... ?

To underline the point that the level of power held by some nurses in Hughes's study was not universally enjoyed, we might look at examples of medical authoritarianism cited in two papers published by nurses in 1987. Smith's portrayal of an incident that took place in a nurse's office vividly illustrates the degree of arrogance that doctors feel able to get away with.

> There, behind the nurse's desk, sits a registrar, while the nurse in charge hovers around attempting to do her work, get at drawers, speak to a relative on the phone and so on. Does the doctor get up and offer her his seat? No, he continues to sit and write up his notes ... The fact that the doctor continues to remain in the nurse's chair shows a lack of respect. It says, albeit indirectly, that she doesn't matter (1987:50).

The following extract from Jones's paper shows just how little influence many nurses continued to have over decisions about care, even in the mid-1980s.

> It seems absurd that post-operative care is carried out not along the lines of a problem-solving approach[5] by the nurses, but on the whims and wishes of the consultants. Take varicose veins. Is it to be legs elevated or legs down? The consultant decides and woe betide the nurse who gets it the wrong way round (1987:59).

These extracts are, of course, not simply pieces of disinterested ethnography. Axes are being ground. Jones's critique is especially interesting, in that it turns medicine's claim to scientific foundation on its head, arguing that it is nurses who use rational methods to solve problems, while doctors act irrationally. The publication of papers such as these demonstrates once again that nurses were no longer prepared to suffer in silence. Both papers conclude with recommendations as to how nurses might go about improving their lot in the future. The fact that nursing empowerment was part of nursing discourse in the 1980s demonstrates that the relationship between nurses and doctors was in a state of flux.[6]

However, it is possible to overstate this point. Melia (1987) in her study of student nurses in the early 1980s noted that students:

> showed little interest in divorcing their work from medicine. They were, in fact, happy to describe certain aspects of patient care as doctors' business ... This willingness to subordinate nursing to medicine was not seen by the students to detract from nursing in any way (1987 180-181).

This lack of enthusiasm for change echoes Hoekelman's contention that in America in the 1970s, there were 'precious few supporters ... among the rank and file of nurses' (1975:1150) for the development of collegial relationships between nurses and doctors. As in the American case, it could be argued 'that the students' view was a realistic one' (Melia 1987:181), given their perception that medical power on the wards was unassailable.

Nursing a problem

Notwithstanding Melia's observations, there is considerable evidence that nursing dissatisfaction with relations with doctors was widespread in the mid-1980s. This can be seen in the results of a study by MacKay (1989) carried out in 1987. Like Hughes, Mackay counsels against easy generalisations. She points out that issues of gender, seniority and specialism will all affect the quality of nurse-doctor interactions. Nevertheless, given that she obtained the views and opinions of 700 nurses in different settings, so we can have a fair degree of confidence in the adequacy of her sample.

Over a third of the nurses interviewed reported that relationships with doctors were not good. Indeed, the degree of arrogance displayed by physicians sometimes astounded nurses:

> One of my first days on the scrub side in theatre, one of the consultants just came up to me and sort of moved me out of the way like a piece of furniture. He didn't acknowledge I was there or anything at all. He just sort of moved me along and I was just totally dumbfounded. I couldn't believe it - I just stood there (1989:42).

Not surprisingly, nurses were far from happy with this sort of behaviour. The overwhelming response of nurse learners to the question of how they thought doctors ought to treat nurses was that they should be more civil and respectful.

However, nurses did not simply blame doctors for the inequality of relations. They recognised that nurses colluded in their own submissiveness. It would seem that Stein's observation that nurses are trained to be subservient still bore some relation to reality in the 1980's:

> I feel that I was always taught to look up at doctors ... and I find it hard to get out of it really. (Enrolled Nurse)
>
> you are taught to respect them in the sense of fearing them and I think that's wrong ... (Staff Nurse) ...
>
> you're trained to be submissive really. You're trained not to bark! (Staff Nurse) (Mackay 1989:44).[7]

However, there was a feeling among senior nurses that the juniors coming up behind them had a different attitude, one which was less tolerant of medical authoritarianism. This was reflected in the (understandable) bemusement of a learner on hearing a story about the behaviour of a nursing sister:

> I was told when I was down in theatre that once, one of the surgeons had forgotten his own clogs so he put some wellingtons on and the sister went out of the theatre because he was in such a bad mood and she hunted high and low for his clogs. She came back with his clogs and she crawled under the table and put them on for him. And I thought is it any wonder that nurses are looked down on by doctors, if the sister will do that? (1989:43).

While this tale has an apocryphal ring to it, its authenticity is not really the issue. Its significance lies in the fact that it indicates that within student nursing culture, subservience to doctors was held up to ridicule. This is a good example of how humour can be used to challenge prevailing social patterns and threaten hierarchy (Douglas 1975).

51

With the introduction of Project 2000 training, it is likely that student nurses will become even more militant. Evidence in support of this thesis comes from Elkan and Robinson's (1991) interim study of the implementation of the reforms, in which they noted that learners were becoming more vocal in asserting their rights.

However, even with such weapons to hand, according to MacKay nurses still had a long way to go. She argues that medical dominance is built in to the health care system within which nurses work. As a result, everything they do is influenced by that dominance. A similar point has been made by Ryan (1989) in response to hopes that Project 2000 students will be capable of changing the system. He argues that inculcation of new ideas into learners is an unrealistic strategy for change because the introduction of anomalous novices will do little to alter current structural arrangements. There are echoes here of Devine's (1978) thesis about the position of nurses in 1970s North America. While the ideology of nurses may be changing, the degree of structural entrenchment that they are faced with makes the prospect of radical change seem remote.

The power to transform

Perhaps these commentators err in placing too much emphasis on the autonomy of structures, and underplaying the capacity of people to transform (rather than simply reproduce) the social structures that they act within (cf Bhaskar 1989b). It may not be the case that new nurses are incapable of altering the status quo, irrespective of their aspirations. New blood **can** generate change.[8] For instance, it has been argued that it was students who were instrumental in bringing in the nursing process (Elkan and Robinson 1991).

Certainly, by the late 1980s a number of commentators were convinced that things had changed, and changed irrevocably.

> one thing is clear: the 'Stepford Nurse\Wife' of yesteryear is gone and has taken with her unquestioning obedience, her hero-worship, her dowry and the camp bed from the duty room. She will not return, in the British health service at least, and there is no point in pining for her in the pages of the *British Medical Journal* (Darbyshire 1987:33-34).

The perception of transformation is not limited to nursing commentators like Darbyshire. Doctors are also feeling the cold winds of change:

> it sometimes seems that with doctors and nurses the rules have been changed, the goal posts moved, the pitch invaded, people sent off for foul play, and someone has run off with the ball. Consequently the doctor-nurse game has had to be abandoned, leaving behind an eerie silence in the stadium (Editorial, *The Lancet*: 1990:218).

The same process has been identified in North America. Stein, in a reconsideration of the doctor-nurse game, notes that physicians' public esteem has deteriorated to the point where they can no longer get away with the pretence of omniscience. Even if they wanted to, nurses are no longer prepared to go along with them.

> The 1967 game was an intricate interaction carefully developed over time in which both players were willing participants. What is happening now is that one of the players (the nurse) has unilaterally decided to stop playing the game (Stein *et al.* 1990:547).

Conclusion

To summarise, it would seem from the evidence cited here that the last two decades have seen changes, though not to the extent that many nurses would wish. Nursing dissatisfaction is the primary driving force behind change, and, as yet, that dissatisfaction has not been assuaged.

Empirical evidence about the position of nurses in the 1980s is not entirely clear. While they do not contain any explicitly contradictory conclusions, the two major studies discussed here (Hughes (1988) and MacKay (1989)) are not entirely in concordance, in that Hughes puts emphasis on the informal powers that nurses enjoy, while MacKay pays more attention to the structural restraints they experience. In Chapter Five, I will attempt to clarify some of this ambiguity by describing the contemporary character of nurse-doctor relationships. However, before discussing the nature of nurse-doctor relations pertaining at present, I will supplement this historical review with an examination of the influence that sociology has had upon the occupational development of nursing.

Notes

1. The rapid adoption of the nursing process in Britain provides a degree of corroboration for Parsons' (1964) neo-evolutionary theory of social development. Parsons argued that social evolution did not need to be repeated in the same form in each society. Evolutionary breakthroughs could be transmitted through the process of cultural diffusion from more advanced societies to those at a lower evolutionary level, allowing less developed societies to evolve rapidly beyond the stage they had got to through their own resources.
2. The prior relationship of opportunity to desire has also been discussed by Elster, using Aesop's fable of the fox which was confronted with grapes out of its grasp as an illustrative framework. Elster notes that:

> The 'sour grapes' mechanism ensures that there is no option outside the opportunity set that is preferred to the most preferred option within it (1989:18).

3. These disarmingly candid admissions that at least one of the purposes of the nursing process was to empower nurses in their relations with doctors are

welcome fare to the sociological commentator. Often the analytic task of sociology is to take the stated aims of actors, and to try to extrapolate from them either unintended consequences or hidden agenda. In this case, the sub-text of the nursing process comes, as it were, from the horse's mouth.

4. Mitchell became something of a straw person, his paper being used by nursing commentators to demonstrate how unfounded the medical response to reasonable nursing demands was. Mitchell's stated beliefs that some nurses saw the nursing process 'as a bid for independence from what they regard as medical domination' (1984:217) and that the process was being used to progressively exclude doctors from nursing affairs, have been portrayed as unreasonable (Clifford 1985) and as examples of sexist bio-reductionism (Wright 1985) While it may well be that Mitchell is guilty of these sins, such guilt cannot be extrapolated from the statements cited by these critics in evidence. Mitchell is simply repeating the claims made previously by enthusiastic (nursing) promoters of nursing independence.

5. The term 'problem solving approach' is an alternative description of the nursing process. It carries with it connotations of practice guided by the results of scientific research, rather than by tradition or personal idiosyncrasy.

6. It might also be noted that the opposite holds. the fact that, up until the 1980s, British nursing journals were largely bereft of such critiques would indicate that medical dominance enjoyed an ideological as well as practical hegemony.

7. Unfortunately, Mackay does not tell us when these nurses were trained. However, the impression gained from the surrounding text is that they were students in the fairly recent past.

8. This argument has been put even more strongly by Kuhn in relation to changes in scientific thought. He contends that change is almost always initiated by new blood:

> Almost always the men who achieve these fundamental inventions of a new paradigm have been either very young or very new to the field whose paradigm they change. And perhaps the point need not have been made explicit, for obviously these are men who, being little committed by prior practice to the traditional rules of normal science, are particularly likely to see that those rules no longer define a playable game and to conceive another set that can replace them (1970:90).

4 Sociology, professionalism and nursing

Introduction

In Chapter Two, I noted that the duality of social structures and individual agents that is implied in the critical realist model entails an over-simplification. Another way of characterising nursing is as an occupational group. As such, it consists of individuals who formulate specific ends and means for it. Because of this fact, an exclusively structural conception is inadequate. However, because the actions of constructed groupings are partially unintended and unforeseen from the perspective of the actors who constitute them (Hannan 1992), a methodologically individualist explanation is also inadequate. Using critical realist terminology, while the strategies of nursing result from intentional actions, they have relational effects upon actors within, and contiguous to, the occupation. It is to these intentional strategies, and their (sometimes unintended) consequences that I now wish to turn.

The occupational strategies of nursing entrepreneurs owe a considerable debt to occupational sociology. As a consequence, if we wish to understand those strategies, we have to appreciate how they articulate with sociological theory. The aims of this chapter are threefold. Firstly, to outline the development of the sociology of professions, and the manner in which sociologists have viewed the occupation of nursing. Secondly, to elucidate the nature of nursing strategies. Thirdly, to show how sociological theories have had an influence upon the strategies adopted by nursing entrepreneurs in their efforts to improve the status of the occupation.

Because this chapter is essentially about the relationship between sociology and nursing, the emphasis given to various strands of sociological thought will reflect their influence on nursing, rather than their more general merit within the corpus of occupational sociology. Thus, for example, because it has had little influence over nursing strategies, the Marxist critique of professions will be given considerably less attention than other critical perspectives.

On the vicissitudes of occupational sociology

The historical trajectory of the sociology of professions has been characterised by what could be called a love-hate relationship between observer and observed. The attitude of sociologists to their subjects has swung violently between whole-hearted sharing of occupational members' understandings at one pole, to disdainful critical detachment at the other (Turner 1985).

Broadly speaking, there have been three phases in sociological opinion. During the first phase, what has often been described as the trait approach to the professions was in the ascendant. This approach was largely uncritical of the professions, accepting unquestioningly the grounds upon which they laid claim to their high occupational status. Yet, at the same time, sociologists pretended to the role of objective commentators. In line with the general retreat of functionalist sociology from the 1960s on, the trait approach fell into disrepute (among sociologists, if not among professionals).

Following the fall of the trait approach, no monolithic sociological consensus emerged to replace it. The second phase involved a bifurcation of analytic focus. The dominant approach during this phase consisted of critical analyses of the professions. Rather than giving credence to the claims made by professionals, critical sociologists concentrated on uncovering the processes through which professions gained so much power. While critical theories were ascendant, they did face challenge from analysts who grounded their position in phenomenological philosophy, and who therefore concentrated on the accounts of professionals themselves.

The third phase has involved the emergence of feminist critiques of the professions. These have incorporated aspects of both wings of the second phase. While critical analysis of the position and role of (male) established professions has continued, feminist observers tend to be supportive of predominantly female occupational groups which aspire to upward status mobility.

Sociology, nursing and the double hermeneutic[1]

The sociology of the professions provides a classic example of the double hermeneutic at work - notwithstanding the critical stance taken by many sociological commentators, there has been a constant two-way communication of understanding between observers and observed.

> The work of sociologists, or of those accepted and cited by sociologists, has played an important part in defining and maintaining a professional culture. But it has not been simply a one-way process. Some statements by professionals addressed to a professional audience have been taken over to become part of the basic corpus of the sociology of the professions (Elliot 1972:139).

Perhaps because of its occupational position, nursing has been more receptive than most groups to sociological insights. Since its inception as an organised occupation, segments within nursing have been engaged in strategies of occupational advancement (Dingwall *et al.* 1988). For several decades now, one of the consequences of this engagement has been that considerable attention has been paid to the pronouncements of occupational sociology. All of the sociological phases mentioned above have had an influence on the manner in which the occupational entrepreneurs of nursing have viewed both the position of their occupation, and the strategies to improve that position.

The first phase: trait theories

Up until the 1970s, the relationship between sociologists and professionals was characterised by mutual support. During this era, the dominant sociological paradigm was the 'trait' approach, which posited that professionalism could be objectively defined through the identification of a fixed set of attributes. One of the earliest and most influential attempts to isolate the defining attributes of a profession was made by Flexner (1915), who listed six criteria which distinguished professions from other occupations. Flexner regarded professional activity as intellectual, learned, practical, taught, internally organised, and motivated by altruism. Since Flexner's statement, there have been innumerable variations on the theme (for example, Carr-Saunders and Wilson 1933; Greenwood 1957) The most obvious problem with these absolutist definitions was that no one definition entirely agreed with another (Cogan 1953; Goode 1960; Millerson 1964).

As well as attempting to isolate the essential attributes of 'professions', the trait approach involved arbitration as to which occupations could claim the honorific title of profession, and which could not (see, for example, Parsons 1939). One of the most influential criteria for the discrimination of professional status was the ability to give the client what the professional decided they needed, rather than having to bow to the clients wishes (see, for example, Marshall 1963; Goode 1966).

Unfortunately for nursing, many trait theorists were unconvinced that the occupation possessed the requisite qualities to deserve the title of profession. Instead, nursing was confined to the limbo of semi-profession.

A good example of this interpretation of nursing's occupational position can be seen in a paper by Katz (1969), which took the core professional trait as being the possession of a specialised body of knowledge. While Katz accepted that nursing had begun to develop a body of knowledge through its adoption of the behavioural sciences, he argued that simple possession was not enough. What was also required was that guardianship of such knowledge was accepted by those outside the profession, most crucially in this case by physicians and hospital administrators. Katz argued that while doctors remained the chief determiners of the kind of knowledge to be used in a health care setting, nursing could not lay claim to the essential attribute of professionalism.

Using a different 'essential' trait, Simpson and Simpson (1969) came to a similar conclusion. They argued that autonomy was the core attribute of professions. They observed that nurses were accountable both to their intra-occupational and extra-occupational superiors - nurse managers and physicians. Echoing Katz, they observed that this high level of control over nurses' work was made possible because they did not possess the weapon of knowledge to resist it. Indeed Simpson and Simpson went further by arguing that, largely because of their feminine attributes, semi-professionals such as nurses tended to lack knowledge, motivation, occupational commitment, and collegiate solidarity. They concluded that hierarchical control over semi-professions was therefore functional for the organisations within which they worked.

According to Simpson and Simpson, the prognosis for the occupational advancement of female semi-professions such as nursing was poor:

> The public is less willing to grant professional autonomy to women than to men, and ... women are less likely than men to develop attitudes favorable to professionalism, because most of them are oriented more toward family roles than toward work roles. So long as our family system and the prevailing attitudes of men and women about feminine sex roles remain essentially as they now are, this basic situation seems unlikely to change (1969:247).

By regarding the possession or the lack of professional qualities as almost immutable, trait theorists provided little comfort for nursing entrepreneurs. The converse of this was that they erected an effective justificatory bastion for the established professions. As we shall see, the anodyne relationship between sociologists of professions and the professions themselves was to become the primary reason for the repudiation of the trait approach. Indeed, questioning of this kind of narrow arbitration first emerged from within the ranks of trait theorists.

Professionalisation theory

The fixed position of trait theory increasingly began to be seen as unsustainably artificial. Such a homogenous model of professionalism was unable to take account of the diversity of occupations which laid claim to the title of profession. This was recognised by some trait theorists, who responded by developing the concept of 'professionalisation'. For example, Vollmer and Mills suggested that:

> the concept of 'profession' be applied only to an abstract model of occupational organization, and that the concept of 'professionalization' be used to refer to the dynamic *process* whereby many occupations can be observed to change certain crucial characteristics in the direction of a 'profession' (1966:vii-viii).

Thus, it was claimed that variations between occupations could be explained by reference to their position on the professionalisation continuum. Wilensky (1964) listed a sequence of events which started with full-time work, and progressed through the establishment of both professional and university education, the creation of a professional organisation, the gaining of legal license, to the final stage of the creation of a code of ethics.

While the dynamic nature of this model made it more flexible than other trait theories, it still involved generalisation from a single observed instance, in this case the professions which emerged in late nineteenth and early twentieth century America. Even the classic professions of Britain failed to adhere to the prescribed sequence. Indeed, in that country, professional power appears to have been attained long before the development of professional knowledge. It was not until the nineteenth century that credentialism replaced spoils and patronage as a means of entering the 'status' professions (Elliott, 1972).

Initially, such inaccuracies did little to compromise the persuasive power of historicised versions of the trait approach. Their strength lay in the fact that they provided ambitious occupations both with the hope of successful advancement, and with a concrete programme by which it was claimed that hope could be realised. Thus, they enabled nursing entrepreneurs to adopt identified professional traits as a yardstick for their occupational projects. For example, in a basic nursing text on sociology, Chapman accepted that:

> it is generally agreed that to be considered as a profession an occupation must have a body of knowledge which is then used as a basis for the practice of a specific skill. There are clearly defined conditions of entry to education and training and there is an examination at the end of the period of education before the appropriate qualification is awarded. Professional organizations control the type of education and standard of examination leading to the professional qualification, and most have a code of ethics backed by a disciplinary procedure to control the activities of their members and protect the client (1977:76).

Descriptions like this were then used to demonstrate that nursing possessed enough of the appropriate requisites to be considered a profession. Thus Hall argued that:

> nursing can make this claim [to professional status] because it reflects certain characteristics of a profession to a very high degree and, in respect of the others, it can be seen to be evolving' (cited Smith 1981:99).

The critique of the trait approach

The rather cosy relationship between sociological observers and their subjects led to considerable disquiet amongst those sociologists who believed that, rather than taking assumptions about the nature of professions for granted, analysis required a critical edge. Trait theory was accused of being:

> contaminated with the ideology and hopes of professional groups rather than an independent assessment of what they achieve. Various occupations play the attribute rating game in an effort to increase their relative standing in the occupational world and to reap the attendant rewards. Sociologists who focus on lists of attributes do not study this process, but participate in it. They have

become the dupe of established professions ... and arbiters of occupations on the make (Roth 1974:17).

Roth and others argued that naive acceptance by trait theorists of professional self-definitions had led to the inclusion of such elements as altruism in many of the checklists, with only a minimum of analysis as to whether it deserved such inclusion. Impressive sounding elements, such as a code of ethics, that were claimed to be exclusive to professions, could be reduced to an obligation to the client which was found in almost all occupations. Even the claim to specialist knowledge was questioned by critics who argued that this sort of knowledge was often irrelevant to day-to-day professional practice (Roth 1974; Rueschmeyer 1964; Wilding 1982).

The second phase: critical theories

In response to the criticisms that the trait approach and its variants were exposed to, there was a swing in the sociology of professions towards a more critical stance. Three broad approaches were developed, linked by the common assumption that the claims of occupations who described themselves as professions should be regarded as problematical.

The neo-Weberian approach

The first major line of analysis focused on the manner by which professionals attained their privileged position. This approach attempted to identify the mechanisms whereby professions actively gained and maintained market control (for example, Jamous and Peloille 1970; Freidson 1970; Parry and Parry 1976 and 1977; Parkin 1979). It was based upon the Weberian concepts of monopolisation and social closure. Weber (1968) saw social closure as a mechanism whereby status groups could shut off access to resources and advantages from other groups. According to Weber, social closure involved the arbitrary identification of certain attributes and their subsequent use as criteria for eligibility to join the privileged group. The criteria could be exclusionary, based on a characteristic of external competitors, or inclusionary, based on qualities of the group 'acquired through upbringing, apprenticeship, and training' (1968:344). Weber observed that one of the most effective criteria in modern society was certification. He argued that demands for certificated educational qualifications as prerequisites for certain occupational positions were not motivated by a thirst for knowledge, 'but rather the desire to limit the supply of candidates for these positions and to monopolize them for the holders of educational patents' (1968:1000).

Interest in Weber's theory of social closure grew during the 1970's and 1980's, with a number of commentators building upon his insights. Parkin (1982) argued that Weber placed too little emphasis upon the role of the state in the process of closure. Parkin insisted that criteria for social closure cannot be arbitrary, but are dependent on the state defining them as appropriate. It is only by persuading state elites to grant them monopoly can professions fully succeed in social closure.

Johnson (1972) noted that in addition and related to monopoly, professions attain their powerful position through the minimisation of supply and the homogenisation of their occupation. These mechanisms are reinforced by the promulgation of ideological justifications for their position in society. Thus professionals promote the image of altruism and ethicality which they claim should only be judged internally. They argue that the high financial rewards they receive is a function not only of the useful work they do but also of the complex skills they possess and the long period of time taken attaining those skills.

In sum, neo-Weberian commentators attempted to identify the mechanisms by which professional status groups have succeeded in maintaining or increasing the privileged social position that they enjoy.

This is not to say that neo-Weberians concentrated solely on processes. Freidson (1970), notably, attempted to identify the defining characteristics of a profession. He rejected the various trait theory definitions, arguing instead that 'a profession is distinct from other occupations in that it has been given the right to control its own work' (1970:71).

The Marxist approach

In contrast to the neo-Weberian emphasis on the attainment of status, Marxist commentators concentrated on the dynamics of the economic base. As a consequence, they tended to regard the actions of professionals as peripheral. The key force in the development of professional power was not seen to be professional self-interest, but the interests of the dominant class - the bourgeoisie (Wilding 1982).

Carchedi's (1977) thesis that professionals act in the interests of capital by maintaining a subservient and disciplined workforce through management and surveillance was representative of this corpus of thought (cf. Johnson 1977; Mellor 1977; Ehrenreich 1978; Navarro 1978).

The radical approach

A third approach accused the professions themselves, rather than capital, of being the source of oppression. This position was exemplified by the writings of Ivan Illich (1977), who identified the basis of professional oppression as being industrialisation and the consequent division of labour, which encouraged the abdication of roles and responsibility. According to Illich, the growth of professionalism entailed the social disablement of individuals. Democratic power was subverted by passive dependence upon professionals. This assertion was supported by Lieberman (1970) who stated that professionalism was inherently a negation of democracy, in that it contained the assumption that lay people were not capable of making decisions that affected their lives. The twin powers of diagnosis and prescription gave professionals a captive market and meant they had the authority to decide when their services should be demanded and by whom. Often these powers were backed up by legal sanction so that people were forced to accept the ministrations of professionals whether they wished to or not.

Illich (1981) accused the medical profession of becoming a major threat to health. Contrary to what he identified as the self-serving myth promoted by doctors, Illich argued that the major determinants of health lay not in the reactive interventions of health professionals, but in the environment. He posited that factors such as diet, housing, hygiene, contraception and working conditions affected health to a far greater degree than the advances of medical science. This assertion was given empirical credence by McKeown's (1976a; 1976b) analysis of the history of mortality rates, which led him to conclude that scientific medical intervention had a minimal role to play in the increase of life-expectancy over the last century.

Illich's argument went further than this. He contended that, rather than simply being inefficacious, much of the impact of medicine had been deleterious to health. By claiming the right to diagnose and treat the illnesses of individuals, doctors diverted attention away from the real causes of disease. According to Illich, this promotion of passive consumption of health care obviated radical and democratic examination of the effects on health of modern industrial societies.

Illich's yearning for a return to mechanical solidarity[2] leaves him open to the charge of indulging in nostalgia for an age that never was. Nevertheless, this does not mean that his ideas have been without influence. As we shall see, some of his sentiments have been adopted by nursing entrepreneurs.

Scientific concept or honorific title?

It should be noted that not all interpretations of professionalism can so easily be put into the conflicting pigeon-holes of functionalism and critical theory. Taking an alternative stand to this dichotomy, some commentators emphasised the importance of actors' perceptions in the understanding of occupational roles and position.

One such commentator was Howard Becker (1971), who argued that the reason for the failure of the trait approach lay in the ambiguities of definition that arose from making the term 'profession' do two different jobs. On the one hand it was being used as a scientific concept, on the other as an honorific title. Becker's solution to this dilemma was to regard professions simply as those occupations which managed to gain the title:

> there is no 'true' profession and no set of characteristics necessarily associated with the title. There are only those work groups commonly regarded as professions and those which are not (1971:92).

Becker was not, however, a radical phenomenologist. While advocating that the sociological focus should be on the 'folk concept' of professionalism, he continued to believe it possible for the sociologist to examine the objective reality of the phenomenon and to compare this reality with the symbol.

Becker's discussion of definition allows us to categorise theorists along three lines: those who attempt to construct objective definitions of the nature of professionalism, those who concentrate on analysis of actors' accounts, and those who attempt to do both.

While trait approaches were fatally flawed in their attempt to conflate objective analysis and honorific arbitration, critical theories were clearer in their analysis. Neo-Weberian critiques, especially, concentrated their efforts upon attempts to objectively identify the nature of occupations that were termed professions.

Both of these positions were criticised by those commentators who felt that the only valid mode of explanation was analysis of the accounts of professionals.

The phenomenology of professions

Robert Dingwall (1977), in his study of health visitor students, provides a good example of the application of phenomenological tenets to the interpretation of occupational position. He contended that, by identifying fundamental criteria which define the essence of professions and applying them as measures of occupations, theories critical of the professions fall into the same trap as trait theories. The logic of both approaches is that:

> a profession is nothing more or less than what some sociologist says it is. He derives his definition from his own members' knowledge of his society or from an inspection of some collection of data. In either case he is basically legislating a social structure by fiat (1977:118).

According to Dingwall, attempts to define what a profession is assume that the term has, or can have, a fixed meaning. Dingwall uses Wittgenstein's argument that words do not have fixed meanings to challenge this assumption. If words do not have rule-governed unequivocal uses, attempts to legislate meaning will inevitably be unsuccessful.

> We cannot, then, define what a profession is. All we can do is elaborate what it appears to mean to use it and to list the occasions on which various elaborations are used (1977:121).

Such an argument should not be taken for granted. The later-Wittgensteinian linguistic philosophy upon which Dingwall relies has been subjected to fierce criticism from commentators such as Ernest Gellner (1968), who argued that it undermines the possibility of intellectual progress through its promotion of arbitrariness and inconsistency at the cost of coherence and unification.

Sociology's continued influence

It might be thought that with critical theories, at least, there would have been a termination of communication between nursing and sociology. On the one hand, the meanings given by nurses to the term 'profession' would be of little concern to sociologists seeking 'objective' criteria. On the other hand, nursing entrepreneurs would be unlikely to find solace in such caustic perspectives.

However, it would seem that the double hermeneutic is more robust than that. One of the most interesting occupational features of nursing has been that while its entrepreneurs have long continued to proclaim the veracity of trait ideology, the practical actions they have simultaneously adopted belies their apparently naive acceptance of the equation propounding that honorific title equals professional status. Indeed, in recent years, the distance between critical examination of professions and the interests of predominantly female occupational groups such as nursing has been considerably narrowed. This development is in no small measure due to the emergence of a feminist sociology of the professions.

The third phase: feminist theories

While accepting many of the basic assumptions of critical theories of the professions, feminist commentators such as Crompton (1987) have asserted the importance of addressing the issue of women's position in society. Crompton notes that:

> Within the corpus of stratification theory neither Marxist nor Weberian class categories are particularly helpful in this respect; both market-derived and labour exploitation theories are gender-blind (1987:424).

This gender-blindness led by default to the unproblematic association of professions with maleness. One of the primary aims of feminist occupational analysis has been to break this association:

> it is necessary to map out a less androcentric terrain within which to locate professions and patriarchy ... The first step on the way to purging analyses of professions of their androcentric bias is to abandon any generic concept of profession and redefine the sociology of professions as the sociological history of occupations as individual, empirical and above all historical cases rather than as specimens of a more general, fixed concept (Witz 1990:675).

Resonances of the relativism advocated by Dingwall can be clearly detected in Witz's statement.[3] However, this emphasis on difference does not entail abandonment of general explanatory models. Both Crompton and Witz advocate the use of neo-Weberian conceptual tools, modified to take account of processes of gendered exclusion, as the most appropriate theoretical approach to the analysis of professions.

The neo-Weberian approach is not the only one that has been utilised by feminist theorists. For example, Celia Davies' analysis, while containing commonalities with those of Witz and Crompton, adopts a more radical approach in her critique of the relationship between professionalism and nursing. Davies argues that traditional professional ideology, because it is inextricably part of masculine culture, has little to offer nurses:

> an advance into old professionalism is an advance into a cul de sac. There is too much in the model that is directly antithetical to what nurses wish to do. Nurses would be better engaged in joining the growing army of those who wish to build a new professionalism from the ashes of the old (1995: 152).

However, even 'new professionalism', with its emphasis on a more democratic relationship with clients (Hugman 1991), is regarded by Davies as containing remnants of the masculine culture of distance and control. As such, it too rests uneasily with the caring ethos of nursing work, an ethos which 'exhibits the humility of interdependence, recognizes the potential contribution of others and seeks to enhance it in a world regarded as more co-operative' (1995:150). The advancement of nursing, then, it not simply a matter of choosing the right occupational strategy; it involves the far wider project of challenging the cultural code of masculinity, which despite the numerical dominance of women, continues to animate the organisation of health care work.

It can be seen that feminist analyses bridge the dichotomy between the critical and phenomenological approaches that emerged in the second phase. This theoretical synthesis has reinforced mutual understanding between nurses and sociologists. For feminist researchers, the experiences of women affected by patriarchal occupational structures are of paramount importance (Du Bois 1983). For women aspiring to improve their occupational position, insights gained from critical analyses of established male professions can be a powerful tool.[4]

Nursing strategies

Being contiguous to an occupational group as powerful as medicine has meant that nursing has long borne the brunt of patriarchal professional dominance. Criticism of the power of medicine can therefore provide nurses with justification for expansion of their occupational autonomy. Nursing entrepreneurs have taken cognisance of critical analyses of professions and adapted their strategies for occupational advancement accordingly.

No longer are nurses prepared simply to claim the honorific title of profession while being denied real occupational power. Predicated upon critiques of (male) professional power, a number of strategies to improve nursing's status have been adopted. As we saw in the previous chapter, starting in North America in the 1960's, and spreading to Europe in the 1970's, there has been growing pressure from nursing theorists to develop the role of the nurse beyond traditional, medically dominated parameters.

According to Salvage (1990), at the core of New Nursing there are two fundamental prescriptions about the appropriate functions of the nurse. The first involves 'adopting a problem-solving approach and using scientifically derived knowledge'. The second entails 'transforming relationships with patients - away from the biomedical model, which views medical intervention as the solution to health problems, towards a holistic approach promoting the patient's active participation in care' (1990:42). Each of these strategies contain strong resonances of the insights developed by critical sociologists (Porter 1992a).

The neo-Weberian strategy

The first of these strategies, the adoption of a problem solving approach, directly addresses the Weberian problematic of monopolisation and social closure. Central to this strategy is the nursing process, which involves the claim that diagnosis and prescription are within the ambit of the nursing role. The importance of this claim rests on the relationship between authority over diagnosis, and professional power (Johnson 1972).

Given that medicine's superordination over nursing has been at least partly due to its monopoly over diagnosis, the importance of successful implementation of the nursing process for the balance of inter-occupational power can be appreciated.

We saw the importance of the process to nursing efforts to alter the balance of power with medicine in Chapter Three. However, while it is the central mechanism in the attainment of a diagnostic role for nurses, it is not the only one. It merely provides a logical framework for nursing actions. There is little in it that could be said to be unique to nurses. It is therefore usually supplemented by a 'nursing model':

> a systematically constructed, scientifically based, and logically related set of concepts which identify the essential components of nursing practice together with the theoretical bases for these concepts and the values required in their use by the practitioner (Riehl and Roy 1980).

Models add flesh to the bones of the process by providing guidance as to when and how the nurse should intervene in health care. To use Salvage's (1990) terminology, nursing models organise 'scientifically derived knowledge' which is then applied using the 'problem solving approach' of the nursing process.

The adoption of the nursing process and nursing models exemplify Witz's (1992) Weberian-feminist characterisation of recent nursing reforms as professionalising dual closure strategies.[5] Not only do they entail challenging the occupational closure enjoyed by medicine, they also enable nurses to engage in an occupational closure of their own. With the enactment of the 1983 Statutory Instruments of the Nurses, Midwives and Health Visitors Act, nurses gained legal recognition for their diagnostic role, thus usurping a previously exclusive medical prerogative. In addition, the law specified that only 'first level' nurses were to be allowed to devise and assess care plans within the ambit of the nursing process, thereby excluding those nurses that did not possess the requisite professional registration.

The passing of this Act is a reminder of Parkin's (1982) argument that support of state elites is an essential prerequisite to successful professional closure. However, as we shall see in Chapter Five, formal powers of diagnosis are not as effective weapons for occupational enhancement as might be thought. We should therefore qualify Parkin's thesis by stating that while state support may be necessary, it is not sufficient.

The anti-professional strategy

Not all of the New Nursing developments fit so neatly into the professional dual closure model. The second New Nursing prescription identified by Salvage (1990) - the promotion of active patient participation in care - is predicated upon a different variant of critical sociological analysis. Incorporation of patients into decision-making processes can be seen as an implicit response to assaults on the power and privileges of established professions, particularly medicine (cf Barrett and Roberts 1978; Ehrenreich 1978; Illich 1981; Kennedy 1981). Illich, for example, argues that doctors disable their clients and that the professional medical monopoly over health care means that patients become passive consumers, unable to take responsibility for the maintenance of their own health.

Nursing proponents of patient involvement in health care appear to concur with this criticism of medicine, while justifying nursing by asserting that the nurse's role is simply to temporarily perform tasks on behalf of patients which, because of their condition, they are unable to do themselves. However, the central task of nursing is seen as returning patients to a state where they are able to perform those tasks autonomously (Orem 1985). This is consistent with Henderson's famous dictum on the role of the nurse:

> The unique function of the nurse is to assist the individual, sick or well, in the performance of those activities contributing to health, or its recovery (or a peaceful death) that he would perform unaided if he had the necessary strength, will, or knowledge, and to do this in such a way as to help him gain independence as rapidly as possible (1966:3).

Moreover, patient autonomy is promoted through the creation of a partnership between nurse and patient. Rather than claiming exclusive professional power over clients, the new nursing theorists advocate joint diagnosis and prescription (for example, Pearson 1988).

There is a certain irony in this strategy of actively involving patients in health care in that it is using an attack on professional power in order to forward the occupational project of nursing. Nevertheless, its logic can be appreciated. By abjuring authority over patients, nursing entrepreneurs are hoping to attain independence from medicine for their occupation.

This shift of authority does not simply entail the replacement of one master by another just as powerful. Admonitions that nurses should accept patients' absolute right to define their own best interests (for example, Murphy and Hunter 1984) ignore the difficulty of removing the unequal power relationship that exists between the sick and their carers (Porter 1988). Patients may well prove to be far more amenable governors of care than doctors ever were.

There are a number of specific means by which the nurse-patient partnership is expressed. Probably most important is primary nursing,[6] which is defined as:

> a system for the distribution of nursing care in which care of one patient is managed for the entire 24-hour day by one nurse who directs and coordinates nurses and other personnel, schedules all tests, procedures, and daily activities for that patient, and cares for that patient personally while on duty (Glanze *et al.* 1986:924).

An extension of primary nursing can be seen in the provisions of the Citizen's Charter for National Health Service clients, which specifies that every hospital patient will be allocated a named nurse (Northern Ireland Health and Personal Social Services 1992).

A more radical manifestation of the attempt to construct an alliance between nurses and patients against the professional power of medicine is found in the nursing role of patient advocacy, which involves:

> informing the patient of his rights in a particular situation, making sure he has all the necessary information to make an informed decision, supporting him in the decision he makes, and protecting and safeguarding his interests (Clark 1982:9).

The rationale for this nursing role is the existence of unequal doctor-patient relationships. It is argued that because the nurse's primary duty is to her patients, she is obliged to speak up on their behalf if they come into conflict with medical staff (Sawyer 1988).

Occupational strategies based on actively involving patients in care directly contradict one of the central tenets of traditional trait theory - that professionals have the right to give clients what professionals decide clients need (Marshall 1963; Goode 1966). Nor, given their inclusive nature, can they be characterised in terms of occupational closure. Thus Salvage argues that the New Nursing reforms should 'be seen as fascinating attempts to construct a new model for occupational authority, rather than as a covert bid for professional status' (1988:519). These attempts are predicated upon the feminist methodological assumption that people should not be treated as objects, but should be regarded as persons, whose subjectivities need to be respected (Stanley and Wise 1983; Hagell 1989).

Ideological hangover

The novelty of new nursing approaches to the occupational role of nurses does not mean that the traditional professionalising model has been left behind; the

68

progression through different phases of occupational conception has not been so neat. While account has been taken of sociological critiques of professions, there remains a strong ideological hangover from the era when sociological analysis and the aspirations of would-be professions were mutually referential. Perhaps because of the anodyne nature of the trait approach, cloaking, as it does, naked occupational competition, its rhetoric continues to be expounded, even though practical strategies have long out-stripped it. It allows nurses the opportunity to flaunt their high-mindedness, and to present it as an ideological justification for their occupational claims (cf. Johnson 1972).[7] Consider, for example, the following statement by a luminary in the British nursing establishment, in which normative ideals about members' values, and analysis of occupational prestige are conflated:

> Professionalism implies a high order of concern and a values system that places concern for others before self interest. The United Kingdom Central Council (UKCC) provides the required legitimacy and authority for nursing, midwifery and health visiting to be called professions. It controls entry, passage and exit through its regulatory system (Emerton 1992:25).

The degree to which this sort of assumption remains part of the shared understanding of nurses should not be underestimated. This occupational self-image continues to be widely disseminated, not least through the medium of training schools. An example of the continuing propagation of trait theory is found in the following extracts from a transcript of my observations of a lecture entitled 'Nursing as a Profession', given to first-year psychiatric nursing students.

The lecture began with the tutor going through a long list of trait theorists, starting with Flexner, listing the attributes that these theorists had legislated as being truly professional. No hint was given that there might be conceptions of professions that lay outside the trait approach, which was given the status of unquestioned truth. Even Freidson was rallied to the cause. The following extract from an overhead transparency was shown to the students in the midst of extracts from the canon of trait theory:

> Freidson argued that the most critical element of a profession is its power to control the terms, conditions and content of its work.

The tutor made no mention of the fact that one of the purposes Freidson's work was to discredit what he saw as the uncritical naiveté of the trait approach. Rather, his identification of the centrality of autonomy was presented as just another step in the incremental acquisition of knowledge about the characteristics of professions.[8]

In addition to presenting trait theory as the given truth, the other main purpose of the lecture seemed to be to demonstrate that nursing had attained the requisite attributes of professionalism. This was evident in the discussion on Freidson's 'definition':

T(F)   Does nursing have this power or who controls it in nursing? [no response] ... Who are we directly responsible to? [no response] ... Who decides what type of training we will have and what conditions there will be?

ST(M)   The Government.

T(F)   Yes, they are important, but who else?

ST(F)   The Board.

T(F)   YES, the national boards and the UKCC. So that would lead us to think that nursing satisfies this one too.

The two themes of presenting trait theory as truth, and of claiming that nursing possessed professional traits, came out even more clearly in the second part of the lecture which consisted of a discussion based around the following list of twelve core attributes, a copy of which was handed out to each of the students:

1) A profession has a unique body of knowledge.

2) A profession produces its own body of knowledge.

3) A profession establishes its own standards and ensures that these standards are enforced.

4) A profession refers to an occupation whose members have a form of higher education.

5) An occupation seen as a profession will be prestigious to its members and to society.

6) A profession is a superior type of occupation.

7) A profession has its own code of conduct and ethical standards.

8) Members of a profession have a responsibility to keep themselves abreast of new developments.

9) A profession is never static, and undertakes research to add continually to the available pool of knowledge.

10) Political development is a necessary pre-requisite for professional development.

11) Members of a profession must achieve strict standards of competence through examination and assessed experience.

12) The function of a profession must be primarily for the benefit of the public.

The tutor described this list to the students in unequivocal terms:

Transcript 4\2
College of Nursing

T(F)   These are the aspects of a profession that make it different from other jobs.

She then went through each attribute to discuss with the students whether nursing possessed it. It was clear she believed that nursing made the grade on all counts. With the exception of two categories (5 and 6), the students agreed with her. However, even when students were dubious about a claim for nursing, the tutor took the line that their objections were unfounded. While she did not directly take on their challenges, she ensured that the discussion quickly got back around to defining nursing as a profession, as the following discussion in relation to Point 6 illustrates:

Transcript 4\3
College of Nursing

ST(F)1 To say that someone's occupation is a profession doesn't mean to say that it's superior. Like, you can't say that a doctor is inevitably superior to a binman.

T(F)   Oh, do you think a binman is a professional? [smug grin which broadens in response to a titter from the class] I'm not saying you don't need skills to be a binman, but why don't we call binmen professionals?

ST(F)2 You don't need special knowledge to be a binman.

T(F)   Yes. They lack the knowledge base of professionals.

In all, the sentiments displayed by this nursing tutor indicate that, at least on an ideological level, trait theories continue to have some use as 'arbiters of occupations on the make' (Roth 1974:17). However, there is still the issue of how such an ideology can sit so comfortably with seemingly contrary practical strategies.

Perhaps discussion about the contradictions inherent in nursing's self-image entails focusing too narrowly on sociological analysis, and neglecting the 'folk concepts' (Becker 1971) of social actors. Evidence from the clinical nurses that were interviewed indicated that while they felt just as comfortable as the nurse tutor in regarding their occupation along the lines of traditional trait theories, they were also happy to affirm the centrality to nursing practice of what I have denoted as anti-professional strategies.

Transcript 4\4
Medical Ward

SP   Would you describe nursing as a profession?

SN(F)   Of course I would.

SP   Why?

SN(F)   Well, it's the sort of job that is a profession. It's got the kind of things that professions have. We've got the UKCC code of ethics. We've got a body of knowledge[9] and so on. I don't think there's any question. We may not get the same sort of pay as the doctors, but I think we're just as professional. More so. Doctors get away with blue murder. They're very wary about disciplining each other. As a nurse, you don't have to do much wrong to find the UKCC's professional conduct committee down on you like a ton of bricks.

SP   If nurses have professional knowledge, do you think that sits well with getting patients involved, if they don't have that knowledge?

SN(F)   Why not? I might have the knowledge, but it's his body, so he should be involved.

SP   But, should a professional not be able to tell somebody what to do for their own good?

SN(F)   No, not at all. At the end of the day, I can give a patient advice, but it would be the opposite of professional to force him.

Once again, we come back to Dingwall's argument that what a profession is will vary according to who is defining it, and all that the sociologist can do is list and elaborate these multifarious definitions. In response to this position, I would note that while it is important to list and elaborate, it is not enough; the sociologist also has a duty to explain social phenomena. In this case, the explanation of the complex occupational self-image of nurses lies in the ideological utility of adopting theories supportive of traditional professions and the practical utility of adopting theories critical of traditional professions.

Conclusion

Notwithstanding the continued adherence to the somewhat worn ideology of the trait approach, it remains the case that nursing theory has been significantly affected by the paradigm shifts that have occurred in occupational sociology. New Nursing roles, with their emphasis both on usurping functions previously monopolised by medicine, and on fostering nurse-patient alliances, cannot be fully understood without taking into account sociological critiques of established professions. Nor can the confidence to turn those critiques to nursing's advantage be appreciated without reference to the increasing influence of feminist thought upon working women.

There is, however, a danger of over-simplifying the relationship between sociology and nursing occupational theory to one of cause and effect. For one thing, such a conception is overly idealist - it fails to take into account the profound influence upon nurses' self-image of the material and social circumstances within which nursing exists, irrespective of sociological theorisations. These circumstances differ greatly according to the location of the nurse. Many of nursing's professionalisers hold senior or academic positions, and therefore are no longer clinical practitioners. While they may well be convinced that the relationship between nursing and medicine needs to be altered to the advantage of the former, there is evidence that many of the rank and file are not of the same mind (Melia 1987). However, as will be seen in what follows, many of the rank and file that I studied were not completely content with their subordinate position.

Secondly, the exchange of ideas between sociology and nursing is not unidirectional - intellectual influences run both ways. Thirdly, there is no guarantee of an immediate, or even swift diffusion of ideas from one intellectual discipline to another. Fourthly, nurses by no means rely exclusively on sociologists for interpretation of their social world, they are quite capable of their own interpretations.

Finally, the significance of gaps in sociological explanations should be appreciated. Second phase critiques were highly cynical in their approach. By treating claims about attributes like ethically governed behaviour and altruism as justificatory gambits, they were unable to address how values such as caring might be central to occupations like nursing. Perhaps this explains the continuing popularity of trait approaches amongst nursing theorists, in that these approaches gave due weight to these values, albeit in an uncritical and sycophantic manner.

The strength of the feminist combination of critique and understanding is that it has gone a considerable way to resolve this dichotomy. It means that commentators can take account of the attributes which nurses believe themselves to possess and which they display in their everyday activities, while at the same time maintaining a critical edge concerning questions of occupational status

Notes

1. 'Double hermeneutic' is a Giddens' neologism, which he defines as:

   The intersection of two frames of meaning as a logically necessary part of social science, the meaningful social world as constituted by lay actors and the metalanguages invented by social scientists; there is a constant 'slippage' from one to the other involved in the practice of social science (1984:374).

2. 'Mechanical solidarity' is the term used by Durkheim (1933) to denote earlier forms of social organisation which were characterised by a low degree of interdependence. With the development of 'organic solidarity', which is characterised by the division of labour through the development of specialised functions, dependence on other individuals increases.

3. Crompton concedes that 'a collapse into relativism' is a danger inherent in such an approach. However, she argues that 'as far as the topic of gender is concerned this potential source of weakness is to be preferred to theories which claim to be all-encompassing but explain little of empirical reality' (1987:424).

4. Not all feminist analyses of occupations provide female workers with optimistic future scenarios. For example, Hearn's (1982) paper on the connection between patriarchy and professionalisation speculates that improvement in the status of predominantly female semi-professions will inevitably be accompanied by their masculinisation. Less deterministically, Crompton (1987) argues that the sex-typing of occupation will be crucial to their status, which will be highly resistant to change.

5. Witz takes the term 'dual closure' from Parkin, who uses it to describe a common strategy of 'semi-professional' occupations aspiring to fuller professional status. It consists of social closure as exclusion: 'the process by which social collectivities seek to maximize rewards by restricting access to resources and opportunities to a limited circle of eligables' (1979:44), and social closure as usurpation, which is 'mounted by a group in response to its outsider status ... [with] the aim of biting into the resources and benefits accruing to dominant groups' (1979:74).

6. This importance was recognised in the north of Ireland in 1990 with the inauguration of the Northern Ireland Primary Nursing Network (Mullholland and Griffiths 1991). the implementation of primary nursing was official policy in the Suburban Hospital where interviews with nurses took place.

7. One should not be too cynical. It could be argued that nursing has a better case for claiming traits such as altruism than almost any other 'profession'. Iris Murdoch (1989) has argued that, apart from teaching, nursing is the only occupation which can evoke spiritual commitment.

8. It might be noted that the co-option of Freidson into the trait camp gives credence to Dingwall's assertion that critics like Freidson have made the same

mistake as trait theorists in attempting to legislate the definition of profession by fiat.

9. This nurse's use of phrases such as 'code of ethics' and 'body of knowledge' is an indication that the lecture on professionalism recounted in Transcripts 4\1-3 was not unique. It is evident that this nurse was also exposed to the argot of the trait approach during her training.

5 Contemporary nurse-doctor relations

Introduction

Having examined the strategies of nursing entrepreneurs, the aim of this chapter is to assess how successful they have been to date in improving the occupational position of nursing. This will be done through description of contemporary nurse-doctor power relations. The nature of relations will be illustrated by data that emerged both from participant observation of interactions between nurses and doctors in the Intensive Care Unit, and from informal interviews with nurses in the Suburban Hospital. In order to operationalise the problem clearly, the data recounted here are largely restricted to the issue of decision making. More subtle manifestations of power differentials are not examined in depth.

Ideal types

Previous attempts to describe the nature of nurse-doctor interaction can be distilled down to four different ideal types. These ideal types will be used as frameworks for organising the data presented here.

Unmitigated subordination

The first ideal type is the traditional view of interaction, which sees the inter-occupational relationship in clear terms of superordination on the part of doctors, and subordination on the part of nurses. This type is consonant with Nightingale's dictum that the sole prerogative to make decisions about who should be a patient, and what should be done for them, lay with doctors, while the nurses' role was limited to assisting their medical superiors and providing a comfortable and hygienic environment (cited Gamarnikow 1978).

Dingwall and McIntosh (1978) have argued that the formative construction of nurse-doctor relations, characterised by severe power differentials, has had lasting

76

consequences. The first ideal type to be examined, then, is one that posits that the 'subservience and second class status of nursing has remained' (1978:107) to such a degree that it involves nurses' unquestioning obedience to medical orders and a complete absence of nursing input into decision making processes. I have termed this type 'unmitigated subordination'. Instances observed where a medical order was given without prior consultation or explanation, where nurses carried out that order without further negotiation and where no alternative explanation could be posited for their apparent subservience, were seen as indicative of unmitigated subservience. Interviews were used to elucidate if nurses themselves felt that they were in a position of unmitigated subordination.

Informal covert decision making

The second ideal type relates to the doctor-nurse game noted by Stein (1967). This involves the pretence of unmitigated subordination, whereby nurses are deferential to doctors and refrain from open disagreement with them, or making direct recommendations or diagnoses, while at the same time attempting to have an input into decision making processes. Situations where nurses made recommendations without appearing to do so by substituting comments about patients' conditions for direct statements; where doctors requested or accepted recommendations in the same fashion and where there was no other feasible explanation for their actions, were categorised as falling under the aegis of what I have termed 'informal covert decision making'. In addition, interviewed nurses were asked whether they recognised this strategy of interaction with doctors, and whether they thought that they themselves used it in their own communications with medical colleagues.

Informal overt decision making

This ideal type emerges from consideration of works such as that by Hughes (1988), which indicated that nurses' influence was greater and more overt than would be expected if the unmitigated subordination or informal covert decision making models were accepted as being universal to all instances of nurse-doctor interaction. However, while the type of intervention into decision making by nurses in Hughes' study was both open and deliberate, it did not enjoy any official sanction. I have therefore called this type 'informal overt decision making'. Instances where there was a breakdown in the deference of nurses to doctors and where they openly involved themselves in decisions about care, but where this involvement was not officially sanctioned, were categorised as belonging to this ideal type. The prevalence of this mode of interaction was also explored in the informal interviews, where nurses were asked how open they felt they were able to be in their contributions to decisions about patient care.

This ideal type corresponds to the new legal status of nursing diagnosis and prescription, following the enactment of the Statutory Instruments of the Nurses, Midwives and Health Visitors Act in 1983. These statutory instruments gave first level nurses the right to devise and assess care plans within the ambit of the nursing process. The aim of the research in this instance was to discover how fully nurses utilised their official prerogative to make decisions about care. This was effected by observing the degree to which nursing process documentation was used as a practical and pertinent tool in the prosecution of nursing care, and by asking nurses how useful they felt the nursing process was, and if it had helped them to develop a diagnostic and prescriptive role that was independent of medicine.

Unmitigated subordination

Observation in the Intensive Care Unit quickly demonstrated that instances of interactions apparently displaying unmitigated subordination were legion. The following are typical examples of what appeared as unproblematic instances of a clear division of power between doctor and nurse:

Transcript 5\1
Intensive Care Unit

SHO(M) His potassium is down to 3.2. Would you change that bag to a litre of normal saline with 40 Kcl?

SN(F)   I'll do it right now.

Transcript 5\2
Intensive Care Unit

SHO(M) [examining observations that had been recorded by the nurse] That tachy [tachycardia] has been up too long. We'd better reduce the dopamine by two.

SN(F)   Down to six?

SHO(M) That'll do.

However, these sequences display an interesting characteristic. On both occasions the doctors took the trouble to explain the reasons for their decisions. If dominance was unmitigated, one would assume that justification for requests such as these would be redundant. This leads to the suspicion that these interactions, rather than displaying unproblematic medical dominance, may be examples of nurses giving their tacit, but considered consent to medical requests.

This impression was reinforced by nurses' interview responses to the question of what they would do if they were given a medical order that they believed to be detrimental to patient well being; for example:

Transcript 5\3
Intensive Care Unit

SP   Would you intervene with medical staff if you thought there was something wrong, or if the patient didn't want to do what they had prescribed, for example discharge?

EN(F)   If there was a definite case, where you could say 'Look, things aren't right for this person to go home'. I think yes, nurses are speaking out more. But I think just a nurse alone decision - no I don't think we could overrule it, but you could certainly put your input into it, yes.

SP   And you wouldn't feel awkward about it?

EN(F)   No, I would not indeed! No, definitely not. I mean, that's what we are all employed for - for the patient. If there weren't any we wouldn't be here.

The statements of nurses in the interviews clearly indicated that they possessed the confidence to speak up and challenge medical orders when they felt the need to do so.

Transcript 5\4
Surgical Ward

SR(F)   I think because nursing staff are becoming more vocal and expressing themselves a bit better that things can only change for the better. They do stick up for their own rights a lot more as well, but they are more vocal from a patient advocate point of view. They are not afraid to speak up on issues that they don't agree with.

Given that doctors frequently justified their requests with explanations as to the reasons for them, and that nurses were quite clear that if they found those reasons unsatisfactory, they would be prepared to challenge decisions, it might be more parsimonious to restrict perceived examples of unmitigated subordination to those instances where medical orders were not accompanied by a justification.

Occasions in the ICU where orders were given without explanation were fairly rare and frequently elicited indications of resentment by the nurses involved, as the following encounter illustrates:

Transcript 5\5
Intensive Care Unit

[Consultant enters the room and stares silently at the monitors that an unconscious patient is attached to for approximately 45 seconds. At first the two nurses in the room stop what they are doing in expectation of some form of communication. After about 20 seconds, however, they return to their work as if the consultant is not there]

CON(M) Inotrope up to ten.

[The consultant turns and leaves the room. The staff nurse that he had focused on while making his statement gives no indication to him that she has heard or taken cognisance of what he has said. After he leaves the room, she turns to her colleague, sighs and shakes her head before going to the drip counter to make the requisite alteration to the rate of infusion].

As was the case in the interaction above, interview accounts indicated that the likelihood of medical orders being given without explanation was closely associated with the seniority of the doctor and the lack of seniority of the nurse.

Transcript 5\6
Intensive Care Unit

SN(F)   As a junior member of staff, if you are going on the ward round, all they would ask you is 'Are they more breathless?'. Even at that, sometimes they just totally ignore you unless you are one of the top level [nursing] staff. All the nurse would be there for is secretarial purposes - pushing the trolley, opening the notes, writing down little bits of messages, occasionally opening a chart and going 'There'. But that would only be the junior level staff, because, you know, we don't know anything. We wouldn't know if the patient has been to the toilet. Though usually its the senior nurses on the round. If I was asked anything which is very rare, I would have the answer there. We went round there about 10 patients and all I was asked the whole time was 'Has she got FOBs [faecal occult blood tests]?'.

It can be seen that while some doctors indulged in authoritarian modes of interaction with their nursing colleagues, these modes were not accepted with equanimity by the nurses they were directed at. Ironically, it may be that it is those nurses who are most likely to experience medical attempts to treat them as unmitigated subordinates, who are also most likely to openly express their resentment towards such strategies. Older nurses often felt uncomfortable with the vociferousness with which some junior nurses responded to what they perceived as medical overbearingness.

Transcript 5\7
Surgical Ward

SN(F)   Nurses on the whole really aren't assertive enough.

EN(F)   The younger ones are. They are a lot more than what we would have been. Sometimes I would think 'Oh my God, listen to her. I wouldn't of dreamt of saying that to a doctor'.[1]

In summary, it can be seen that instances of unmitigated subordination occur much less frequently than might have appeared to be the case at first glance. When they do occur, they often involve interactions between senior medical and junior nursing staff. Junior nurses do not accept the validity of adopting unmitigated subordinate roles, and are on occasion prepared to challenge medical attempts to adopt such positions.

Informal covert decision making

The next form of interaction to be addressed is that which Stein called the doctor-nurse game, and which I, rather more laboriously, term informal covert decision making. This involves nurses surrogating statements about patients' conditions for open recommendations.

After analysing the results of participant observation in the Intensive Care Unit, I was left in somewhat of a quandary as to whether the doctor-nurse game was being played or not. As with the category of unmitigated subordination, first appearances seemed to suggest that it was a frequently used mode of communication, as the following example illustrates:

Transcript 5\8
Intensive Care Unit

SHO(M) Everything OK?

SN(M)   His pain isn't well controlled

SHO(M) Yes, I think he could well do with another two mls per hour of morphine.

SN(M)   Fine.

What led me to suspect that there were additional complexities within interactions such as this was the affirmative with which the doctor prefaced his order with. The pattern of his speech was more appropriate as a response to a suggestion than to a simple statement. If one discounts the possibility of communicative incompetence, one is led to the conclusion that the doctor is not greatly interested in maintaining the masquerade of omniscience, in that he is prepared to openly recognise the existence of an implicit suggestion.

My suspicion was reinforced when I compared this interaction to a similar one on the subject of pain control which occurred several days before, and which included the same actors:

Transcript 5\9
Intensive Care Unit

SN(M) [To doctor] Forename!

SHO(M) Yea?

SN(M) Mr Surname's still in pain. Shall I increase his morphine by a couple of notches?

SHO(M) Sure.

This led me to ask why two actors who were capable of communicating in such an open fashion at one point, with the nurse making an overt suggestion about an alteration in care, should later feel it necessary to take the trouble to indulge in an elaborate game in order to communicate almost identical information. I could not find any reason as to why deference was required in one situation and not in the other, and so concluded that, in these instances at least, a solution should be sought outside the confines of the doctor-nurse game. I suggest that what appears to be deference in the former transcript is in fact simply shorthand. As is recognised by Stein in his formulation of the doctor-nurse game, and indicated by the doctor's response, the explicit identification of a problem carries with it an implicit suggestion as to its solution. Given the specificity of the problem and the situation, possible solutions in this instance were reduced to a binary alternative: either to give more morphine or not to. Both actors understood this and realised that the other understood as well, so there was little information to be gained by the nurse openly spelling out his suggestion. The fact that both forms of interaction recorded above were used frequently throughout the ICU, with little indication that the choice of either affected the quality of interaction, suggests that the doctor-nurse game cannot explain all instances of implicit nurse-doctor communication.

Evidence gained from the interviews is also rather ambiguous, but on balance would suggest that reliance on informal covert decision making has been decreasing over time, and that nurses are now prepared to express their recommendations in a more direct manner than used to be the case. This is not to say that the doctor-nurse game has been totally abandoned, as this junior Staff Nurse's response demonstrates:

Transcript 5\10
Medical Ward

SP   How much responsibility do you think you take in decision making?

SN(F)   I would say its more prompting. Say, maybe in an arrest situation, something like that, you would say 'Would you like this?' If they aren't making the decision very quickly, whenever you've been here, you know the regime for things and you would say 'Would you like whatever?'. But they are taking the final decision whether they want it or not. Personally I wouldn't say anything directly. I would like them to make the decision and make sure they knew they were making the decision. They're accountable. It is a doctor's decision.

The striking thing about this statement is the situational example that the nurse gives - decision making during a cardiac arrest. It might be supposed that of all situations, this is the one where the etiquette of deference would be most likely to be dispensed with, given the paramount importance of swift response. The bizarre image conjured up by this account is a reminder of just how powerful social *mores* can be. However, notwithstanding the fact that informal covert decision making strategies are still used, even in the most inappropriate of circumstances, most nurses interviewed were clear that nurses now had the legitimate opportunity to openly involve themselves in decision making.

Transcript 5\11
Surgical Ward

SR(F)   It has changed - before we wouldn't have done that - we would have skirted round the issues and dropped a few subtle hints and tutted and carried on ... but now - I'm not saying it is the ward sisters that are doing that - it is the primary nurses who are doing that and they are making their feelings known - that they have feelings and they are speaking out.

Transcript 5\12
Surgical Ward

EN(F)   Ten years ago, I might have been reluctant to speak out to them, whereas now, with experience, you know , you just say 'No, you can't do that, you should do...' or 'would you not consider' Then they'll listen, but only the junior doctors. Though the new consultant appears to be very open. Whereas before on the ward rounds, the nurses weren't acknowledged, whereas now this new consultant and even the SHOs would actually turn and say to you a lot more now than what they used to. They would always ask your opinion.

My evidence that reliance on informal covert decision making strategies has decreased is consonant with Stein *et. al.*'s (1990) description of the collapse of the doctor-nurse game since Stein first published his paper in 1967. However, Stein *et. al.* attribute changes exclusively to alterations in the attitudes and actions of nurses. The impression gained from the second transcript above is that it is not simply a matter of nurses forcing changes. Instead, there would appear to be a willingness on the part of many younger doctors to see at least some degree of democratisation in the relationship. This impression is reinforced by the comments of other nurses.

Transcript 5\13
Surgical Ward

SR(F) I must say that the medical staff - not just the consultants, the SHOs down - if they didn't allow us the climate to do that [speak out], it would be very difficult. On their part they do listen to us. They know that we're here all the time and probably have more contact with the patients and do have some knowledge. They are not treating us as being stupid anymore, like they used to. Having said that I think the calibre of nurse now has improved. I think nurses are not afraid to speak out and they are looking to extend their knowledge.

Doctors' new found respect for nursing opinion need not be interpreted as another instance of fabled medical altruism - there are good functional reasons why doctors should abandon the doctor-nurse game. As Stein noted, its major disadvantage 'is its inhibitory effect on open dialogue which is stifling and anti-intellectual' (1967:703). As the Sister above points out, the large amounts of useful information that nurses possess, not least by dint of being in constant contact with their patients, can be far more efficiently tapped by means of open and direct communication. In a climate where medicine has lost some of its aura of public respect and is required to justify itself more and more (Stein *et al.* 1990), it can no longer afford the luxury of strategies as crassly inefficient as the doctor-nurse game, when the only justification for such strategies is the generation and maintenance of status.

It would be a mistake to overemphasise the medical contribution to the development of more open communication. Not all doctors are happy about embracing new ways of relating. However, even when doctors prove resistant to the freeing up of inter-occupational dialogue, nurses are still often prepared to make their views known, regardless of medical preconceptions about appropriate discursive practices.

SN(F)   Sometimes the consultants ... don't really want to listen very much to you ... They listen to the information you're giving, but you might have one view of what the patient might need or want, and you voice your opinion, but the consultant has got his own idea and, regardless really of what you are saying, at the end of the day, he's going to stick to his decision I think.

SP   Knowing that with consultants, would you make open recommendations?

SN(F)   I would be the sort of person that just said anyway. I wouldn't make blasé remarks or comments, but if I feel the patient needs something or its important to the patient's care, well, I will obviously say it. [Consultant surgeon] just thinks I'm 'a very cheeky gal' and that just says it all [laughs].

While the extreme obfuscations of the doctor-nurse game may be coming increasingly anachronistic, this does not mean that nurses can abandon altogether niceties of interactive performance designed to smooth the professional feathers of their medical colleagues:

Transcript 5\15
Medical Ward

SP   Do instances of friction between nurses and doctors occur?

SN(F)   I think there can be times, it depends on the way that you say things to the doctors. I think its like any of us - if anyone comes up to you and are cheeky, you would just get on your high horse and don't do what they want you to do. Whereas if you approach the doctors in a nice way, they would be more likely to agree with you. I suppose there are more nurses who feel that they would know a wee bit more than the doctors, especially newly qualified nurses, and maybe some of the nurses would go up to them and say 'Look, do you really think you should do that?' and then they would feel 'Well, I'm the doctor here'. It just depends on their attitude. I doesn't happen all that often - very infrequently, though some nurses would take it further than they used to, though it can be counterproductive. Its the way you approach them. You have to do it in such a way that you're not trying to tell them their job, but still try and get over your opinion.

It can be seen from this statement that abandonment of the doctor-nurse game does not entail abandonment of deference. Indeed, the cost of failing to be sufficiently deferential can be that it triggers a recidivistic response in doctors, who attempt to return the offending nurse to a position of unmitigated subordination. To overstep the mark is to risk being reminded that the nurse-doctor relationship is far from equal.

In summary, while the doctor-nurse game is still played by some nurses and doctors, full blown manifestations of it are largely confined to interactions involving rather traditionalist senior medical staff, or junior nursing staff who lack confidence about their position. However, while nurses are no longer expected to masquerade as being incapable of decision making, they are often still expected by doctors to be deferential, and, in cases of disagreement, to acquiesce to medical decisions. Not all nurses are prepared to remain so reverential. As we shall see, many, especially those in senior positions, are able and prepared to push the boundaries of nurse-doctor interaction considerably further.

Informal overt decision making

Nurses do not appear to feel constrained from frequently making overt suggestions about care. Indeed, in many cases, nursing input into decisions is not limited to suggestions that can be accepted or rejected by their medical colleagues. Senior nurses, especially, are prepared to argue in support of their proposed line of action in the face of attempted rejection by doctors, as the following interaction recorded in the ICU demonstrates:

Transcript 5\16
Intensive Care Unit

SN(M)   What lines shall I take out before he goes to the ward?

SR(F)   What has he got?

SN(M)   Two peripheral and a three-lumen central.

SR(F)   You can put the morphine pump and the saline through two of the central lumen and scrap the peripherals.

SHO(F) How about using the peripherals instead, so the poor houseman up there can take bloods from them?

SR(F)   Hmm ... it's more important to keep the central line going.

SHO(F) Could you not put one line through the central and one through a peripheral?

SR(F)   That would be a bit awkward for transferring him to the ward bed.

SHO(F) Oh well, whatever you think. [exits]

SN(M)   Well, which lines will it be?

SR(F)   He's not going up there with lines hanging out of every available limb.
Take one of the peripherals out, bung the other and stick the lines
through the central.

Not only are nurses often prepared to assert themselves in fairly loose
conversational situations such as that recorded above, but if they do not agree with
direct medical orders about patient care, they have the opportunity to voice their
misgivings.

Transcript 5\17
Intensive Care Unit

SHO(M) Could you take down Mrs Surname's morphine pump please? She's
been on it long enough now.

SN(F)   I don't think she's ready for that yet. We've been trying to reduce it
today, but every time we do, you can see the pain breaking through.

SHO(M) OK. If you can try and reduce it over the next 24 hours, we'll think
about it again tomorrow.

What is striking about this interaction is the similarity of the opening sequence to
the transcribed examples of what appeared to be unmitigated subordination
(Transcripts 5\1 and 2). The fact that the conversation above takes a direction that
shows anything but subordination reinforces the impression that when nurses act on
medical orders without comment, they are displaying implicit agreement rather than
meek subordination. Indeed, interactions were noted where the apparent format of
unmitigated subordination occurred with the doctor in the 'subordinate' role.

Transcript 5\18
Intensive Care Unit

SHO(F) How's he doing?

SN(F)   He's been spiking a temp [temperature] since 4 O'clock this morning.
You'll need to take some blood cultures.

SHO(F) OK. No problem.

SN(F)   Thanks.

Occasional instances were noted where nurses took decisions which by law were the sole prerogative of medical practitioners, as another morphine anecdote illustrates:

Transcript 5\19
Intensive Care Unit

SR(F)   Did I tell you that we stopped his morphine at midnight?

SHO(F) No, I don't think so.

SR(F)   He was too doped.

SHO(F) That's grand. We'll keep it down unless he gets sore again.

This is a good example of how the exigencies of work described by Hughes (1988) can operate to increase nursing input into decision making. In this case, because of the desire to sleep at night while they are on call, doctors tend to be extraordinarily sanguine when nurses flout the normal rules governing the division of labour when it means they are not disturbed.

It can be seen that, despite the uneven ground rules for interaction, many nurses in many situations have managed to leave behind the 'Victorian ethos' of medical supe-riority, and are expecting to participate in dialogue governed by rationality rather than traditional authority. Perhaps this self-confidence can be most clearly seen in the steady withdrawal of nurses from the handmaiden activities that were once expected of them. This process is outlined by a nurse of 15 years experience:

Transcript 5\20
Medical Ward

SN(F)   [Nurses are] no longer going to be regarded as the doctors' handmaidens. And I think doctors even, the new doctors coming out, are more approachable. They don't really, a lot of them anyway, don't expect you to run after them and things like that. You do get the odd one who does.

SP   How would you react to them? Would you run?

SN(F)   No, you would discretely say to them 'Really, that's not our job' or 'Really, we're not here to run after you'. We would show them where everything is and show them where to put things, and things like that, and sort of discretely try and get them into the way of thinking that we are no longer here to tidy up after them and things like that. If they still don't learn, we would get Sister to have a word in their ear. You try not to run after them. You try to make them realise that you're here to look after the patients and to carry out their care, not to run after them. That's a big change. Gone are the days where you made them coffee and things like that. You don't do that any longer.

In summary, the evidence presented here suggests that informal overt decision making is a widely practised nursing strategy, used with differing degrees of assertiveness depending on the situation and the status of the nurse and doctor involved.

Formal overt decision making

The empirical evidence about the degree to which nurses utilised the nursing process as a method of formal decision making is somewhat contradictory. Many of the nurses from the Suburban Hospital reported that the nursing process was a useful innovation. However, observation of nurses in the Intensive Care Unit provided little indication that it was being significantly utilised.

Given that the nursing process is the only officially sanctioned and, indeed, compulsory form of nursing decision making, it was surprising to discover that it was profoundly under-used in the ICU. On the admission of each patient, considerable time, often in excess of an hour, was spent listing each of their problems and what was to be done about them. Much of this took the form of mundane routine, with the same formulae being painstakingly written out in long hand on every occasion.

Given the amount of effort expended to formulate this information, it was surprising to discover that it was subsequently almost totally ignored by nurses. It was brought out three times in every 24-hour cycle in order that the compulsory reports could be written. Apart from these occasions, it was rarely consulted, with almost all information being transmitted orally. It seems that it functioned more as a legal document than as an aid to nursing care.

Given these results from participant observation of nurses in the Intensive Care Unit, it was surprising to discover that most of the Suburban Hospital nurses interviewed thought that the nursing process was a useful tool. While the perennial clinical nursing complaint that the process entailed too much paperwork, and filling it in meant that nurses lost valuable clinical contact time was voiced on a number of occasions, almost all nurses asked were unequivocal that, despite its shortcomings, the nursing process was an effective way of organising care.

Transcript 5\21
Medical Ward

SP   Do you think the nursing process is useful?

SN(F)   It's useful for getting all the information that you need and carrying out a plan of care in a routine fashion. OK, it may be routine but at least everything is covered. It's not routine care, it's routine planning. But everything's covered, you get an overall view of the patient; what you're doing, what their needs are, and support when they are going home. You know, how they've coped since the day of admission and how they're coping throughout the hospital, and what things are going to be like at home.

Transcript 5\22
Medical Ward

SP   Do you think that the process is useful?

SN(F)   Yes, I think it is because I think it makes us aware what problems the patient has ... Not just to look at a patient, and say that patient's in with angina, so you're treating their chest pain. But actually to sit down and break down what problems that patient has, such as a venflon,[2] such as anxiety, such as health education, you're not actually just treating them as a chest pain, you're treating them as a whole person. So I feel, yes. Again, if you have students coming on to the ward. If they're able to read those care plans, it gets them into the way of what we're looking for with these patients. So, yes, I think it keeps everybody on their toes, aware of what problems these individual patients have.

What was striking, however, was that while most Suburban Hospital nurses found the process useful, they had little sense of it being used as a tool for independent diagnosis and planning.

Transcript 5\23
Surgical Ward

SP   Would there be any areas within the nursing process where you would feel that it is a nursing remit completely, that it is a nursing diagnosis and there is no reason to consult the medical staff?

SR(F)   It is a very tricky area ... Pressure sores? I can give you an example, if we said to the consultant 'Look, Mr So-and-So has a pressure sore', he would turn round and say to you 'What are you putting on it?' He wouldn't think of prescribing anything, which is fair enough. But we wouldn't prescribe. The primary nurse would decide what she felt would be best on it. She would decide that in consultation with the other nurses and with myself and we come to a decision as to what was

90

going on it. We would then - I suppose this is being sneaky, but - we would then ask the doctor, 'Look, we think such and such a thing is needed for this sore or whatever. Would you write that up?' We wouldn't put it on without having it written up, but we would have decided.

The transcript above indicates that as a tool for independent diagnosis and planning, the nursing process has not been entirely successful, in this context at least. While it might pretend to formal diagnostic and prescriptive status, in reality the process has little formal authority, in that the proposed actions emerging from it have no institutional mandate until they have been given the blessing of doctors. While the process is used as a framework for *de facto* decision making, it has not delivered *de jure* autonomy.

When pressed, the consensus amongst the nurses was that doctors still maintained a fairly tight grip of formal control over all aspects of physical care. Indeed, it was pointed out to me that administrators' fears about what they perceived as an increasingly litigious health service clientele had led them to progressively introduce rules which had the effect of reducing nurses' opportunities for carrying out physical interventions without medical authorisation. One nurse complained to me that according to hospital regulations she was now forbidden to apply moisturising lotion to a patient with chapped hands unless the lotion had been medically prescribed.

The one area where it did seem that the nursing process afforded nurses autonomy was that of psychological care.

Transcript 5\24
Medical Ward

SP   Has it [the nursing process] introduced diagnosis?

SN(F)   I think you do make a diagnosis. You get to know your patient as a whole with it. I think that its good in that way. And you can take out their individual problems and you can decide the care for them. I think it does give you that wee bit of power.

SP   Can you give me an example?

SN(F)   Anxiety is one of the things. I don't think doctors take into consideration how anxious a person is, whereas we can. We can get to talk to them and see how anxious they are. We can see where they need a lot of information about their care and things like that there, their diagnosis and things like that. I think that area is important. And that would be done entirely on a nursing basis.

It appears that areas of care and treatment which are valued by doctors remain firmly within their grasp. It is only in those areas which medicine tends not to regard as highly important that nursing has space to develop.

In all, the effects of the nursing process do not appear to have been as far reaching as its progenitors might have hoped for. Firstly, it would seem that the enthusiasm with which it is adopted varies markedly between different institutions. Secondly, even in institutions where there appears to be a genuine commitment to full implementation of the process, many of the decisions nominally under its ambit remain within formal control of medicine.

To date, the introduction of a formal decision making capacity has had considerably less impact upon the position of nurses than the informal strategies that they appear to be increasingly adopting. However, there are exceptions to this rule. As we shall see in Chapter Eight, the setting up of a Nursing Development Unit in the Suburban Hospital provides a good example of just how effective formal reforms can be in altering the balance of power between nurses and doctors, if they provide an environment which nurses find conducive to asserting their autonomy.

Conclusion

Even when the subtleties of interaction are forced into four general types, the resulting picture remains a complex one. All four ideal typical modes of interaction were manifested in the research data. Often different types were displayed at different times by the same person. As a result, there can be no simple answer to the question 'How do contemporary nurses interact with their medical colleagues?'. Nevertheless, it is possible to discern a reasonably clear picture of the state of play. Three broad conclusions can be drawn.

Firstly, the continued occasional use of both unmitigated subordination and informal covert decision making bear testament to Trotsky's dictum that throughout history, the mind limps after reality. The imprint of earlier social formations and divisions of labour continue to haunt the present.

Secondly, it is apparent that the present division of labour does involve a qualitative change (or at least a process in which change is occurring). The balance has moved in favour of rational dialogue at a cost to discourse based upon the unquestioned power bestowed by occupational status. This shift is evidenced by the frequent and uninhibited adoption of overt informal decision making by many nurses.

Thirdly, while nurses may feel better able to make their voices heard, the effectiveness of those voices is still stringently limited by the powers that remain in the hands of doctors. In terms of formal power, despite the implementation of the nursing process, in many cases there is little evidence of significant nursing advancement.[3] However, it would be unwise to conclude that formal advancement had reached a dead end. A more judicious conclusion would be that the growth of formal nursing power is characterised by uneven development.

The contemporary pattern of nurse-doctor power relations, as manifest in decision making, is one where it is increasingly expected by all parties (to greater or lesser degrees) that communication should be free from obfuscating etiquette. However, while decision making may now be done in the open, with nurses feeling it is their right to participate, both sides are also well aware that, in the last instance, the balance of power still remains firmly in the hands of doctors.

Nevertheless, relations have changed dramatically over time, as the memories of a staff nurse who had been working since the early 1960s in the Suburban Hospital demonstrate:

Transcript 5\25
Surgical Ward

SP   Have the way doctors and nurses relate to each other changed at all since you started?

SN(F)   Oh, that has changed. When I started nursing - I was reared in the country and when the doctor was coming to the house, it was polished from top to bottom and the best linen and hand towels were got out and all this fuss went on and when I started nursing, it was still in nursing. The ward had to be perfect. The wheels had to be turned a proper way when the doctors came on the ward round and they were 'sirs' and 'misters' and all this and you as a student nurse were there as everybody's dogsbody at that stage. But even as you got up as a staff nurse, they were very much the 'sir'.

It can be seen from this transcript that the efforts of nursing entrepreneurs to improve the status of their occupation have met with some success. However, it would a commission of what Bhaskar (1989a) calls the error of voluntarism to explain changes in the position of nurses exclusively in terms of the agency of influential nurses. Nurses, in common with all other human agents, live within the ambit of social structures, which both constrain and enable their actions. It is to the explication of the influence of structures upon nurse-doctor power relations that the next section is dedicated.

Notes

1. This transcript and the one previous to it give us some insight into the issue discussed in Chapter Three as to whether newly recruited nurses can be effective change agents. It would seem that two countervailing currents are at work. On the one hand, because they are junior, medical staff feel they should be more subservient. On the other hand, because they are newly arrived in nursing, they have not been fully inculcated with traditional norms of interaction, and have enjoyed a more empowering form of education.

2. 'Venflon' is the tradename for a type of intravenous cannula.
3. Giddens (1976) has argued that the processes of structuration involve an interplay of meanings, norms and power. In this case, it might be observed that while the meanings and norms involved in inter-occupational relations have significantly altered, formal power has not because it is embedded in the relatively immutable structure of state-sanctioned legality.

Part Three
EXPLAINING NURSE-DOCTOR RELATIONS

6 Patriarchy

Introduction

It will be remembered that one of the central methodological approaches that I wish to adopt in this research is the application of critical realism as an underlabouring philosophy. In the previous part I described the characteristics, both historical and contemporary, of nurse-doctor relations. In this part, I hope to identify and elaborate on the social factors which play a part in forming those relations.

In line with the tenets of critical realism, three of the chapters in this part will deal with structural issues - patriarchy, racism and capitalism. However, before discussing these areas, it is important to underline the limited nature of critical realism. Bhaskar is at pains to emphasise that:

> Realism is not, nor does it license, either a set of substantive analyses or a set of practical policies. Rather it provides a set of perspectives on society (and nature) and on how to understand them. It is not a substitute for, but rather helps to guide, empirically controlled investigations into the structures generating social phenomena (1989a:3).

For one thing, we cannot look to critical realism to tell us which structural mechanisms are at play in any specific instance. That can only be done through both the formulation of synthetic a priori hypotheses about the sort of structures that would be required to exist for regular phenomena to occur, and the subsequent gathering of empirical evidence to confirm the existence and illuminate the mechanisms of those structures.

Similarly, critical realism cannot tell us which of a multiplicity of structures has the most profound influence upon a social phenomenon, though it does indicate that such an exercise is both possible and desirable.

> Social phenomena ... are the product of a plurality of structures. But such structures may be hierarchically ranked in terms of their explanatory

importance. Such an approach allows us to avoid the pitfalls of both crude determinism (for example, of an economic reductionist sort) and undifferentiated eclecticism (1989a:3).

In response to the issue of which structural mechanisms were at play in this instance, I concurred with commentators such as Williams (1989) that the divisions of gender, 'race' and class are the most significant in contemporary Western societies, and would therefore be of most significance in this social setting.[1] My justification for doing so lay in my observation of the stark gender division of labour in formal health care; in the isolation of members of racialised groups to a specific occupation, namely medicine; and in the fact that, even though they were state employees, the activities of doctors and nurses occurred within a capitalist economic system.

Another problem is how these structural inequalities should be ranked in terms of their salience to the situation being examined. The choice of which structural mechanism should be regarded as dominant was not difficult. As Game and Pringle observe, 'The primary division of labour in health represents a sexual division in its starkest form, namely that between male medicine and female nursing' (1984:94).

While the prioritisation of patriarchal relations in this specific social situation is justified, it should not be assumed that the three structural elements that have been chosen are discrete entities, operating independently of each other. Rather, each acts to partially constitute the others. Thus,

> analysis of gender relations in contemporary western societies is constituted by a system of patriarchal relations in articulation with a system of capitalist relations ... The actual pattern of gender inequality should be seen as the outcome of the interaction of these two systems together with that of racism (Walby 1986:50).

Patriarchy and nursing

The crucial importance of gender relations in explaining the position of nurses *vis-à-vis* doctors is reflected in the frequency with which it is cited in the literature (for example, Stein 1978 [1967]; Hoekelman 1975; Kalisch and Kalisch 1982a [1977]; Lovell 1982; Game and Pringle 1984; Wright 1985; Keddy *et al.* 1986; Darbyshire 1987; Jones 1987; Smith 1987; Mackay 1989; Stein *et al.* 1990; Davies 1995). Because those gender relations entail the exploitation of women by men, they can be described as patriarchal (Walby 1986). In addition, because patriarchy involves enduring relations between societal positions of actors, and because it lies behind, and affects, manifest interactions, it falls within the critical realist criteria for a structural mechanism (Bhaskar 1989a). This is not to say that patriarchy is a universal and immutable system. The form that gender relations take results from their maintenance or transformation by human action (Crompton and Sanderson 1990). One of the primary points that I wish to make in this chapter is that gender relations have changed, and are continuing to change, largely as the result of women's actions.

Patriarchy affects nursing in five interconnected ways. Firstly, because nursing is popularly seen as mundane 'women's work', analogous to the tasks involved in domestic labour, it is devalued (Abbott and Wallace 1990). Secondly, because nursing is situated within a stark sexual division of labour alongside the predominantly male occupation of medicine, gender relations animate inter-occupational inequalities (Gamarnikow 1978). Thirdly, because the culture of organised health care is inherently masculine, women working in that culture are placed in the position of the inferior 'other' (Davies 1995). Fourthly, because nurses' sexuality is subject to misogynous stereotypification, their occupational subordination is further overdetermined (Muff 1982). Fifthly, with the development of a predominantly male managerial elite, gender inequalities are increasingly becoming an issue within nursing (Hearn 1982; Carpenter 1977 and 1978).

The purpose of this chapter is to illuminate how the social structure of patriarchy affects the occupational position of nurses. Four major substantive areas are addressed: firstly, how gender affects power relations between doctors and nurses; secondly, how gender affects power relations between male and female nurses; thirdly, how nurses interpret issues of gender, and finally, how sexual stereotyping affects relations between doctors and nurses.

The sexual division of labour

The most striking difference in the composition of medicine and nursing is sex. Since its rise as an organised profession, medicine has been a predominantly male occupation while nursing has long been regarded as one of the archetypal female occupations. Examining the nineteenth century formation of occupational relationships between nurses and doctors, Gamarnikow has argued that they can be equated with Victorian family relationships.

> This ideological reconstruction of interprofessional relations and their transformation into male-female relations operated by representing the nurse-doctor-patient triad as essentially homologous to the family structure. Thus nurse-doctor relations came to be seen basically as male-female relations and the patient became the 'child' The equation ... provided the ideological space for turning nurses into 'mothers' and doctors into 'fathers' (1978:110).

Doctors, being invested with the 'rule of the father', possessed the sole right to decide who should be defined as a patient, while nurses in their mothering role were expected to be both subordinate to the patriarch, and caring towards the patient.

Dingwall and McIntosh (1978) have argued that this type of patriarchal relation continues to animate occupational relations:

The Victorian ethos of male superiority reinforced the nurses' deferential attitudes to doctors far into the twentieth century, and the idea of a colleague relationship is a relatively new concept ... Despite the pressure for greater status, and influence at a policy making level, the subservience and second class status of nursing has remained (1978:107).[2]

To summarise, occupational relations between nurses and doctors have, since their outset in the nineteenth century, been structured by patriarchy. The specific formation of patriarchal relations in this instance resulted from a complex interpolation of domestic and occupational gender inequalities, which in turn were connected by the ideology of sex roles.

Intra-occupational inequalities

Female disadvantage is not limited to differences between these occupations, it is equally notable within them. Despite recent increases in the number of women entering medical schools, the profession remains firmly in the hands of men.[3] This is evidenced by vertical segregation within the occupation which means that women occupy proportionately far fewer senior posts than their male counterparts, and also by horizontal segregation. In general surgery for example, less than 1 per cent of consultants are female. Women tend to be concentrated in specialities such as child and adolescent psychiatry (Oliver and Walford 1991).

Numerically, male entry into nursing has been considerably less significant than female entry into medicine. In 1987, fewer than 10 per cent of nurses in Britain were men (Gaze 1987). The fate of this small male minority has, however, been considerably more auspicious than that of its female counterpart in medicine. Men have been able to exploit the patriarchally subordinated position of women to leapfrog over their female colleagues in nursing's career race (*cf.* Crompton and Jones 1984 on male advantage in clerical work). With the introduction of an industrially modelled line management system following the Salmon Report (1966), men came to dominate the management of both nursing practice and education, to the point where by 1987 they held over 50 per cent of chief nurse and director of nurse education posts in Britain (Gaze 1987). There was an implicit sexism in the Salmon Report; it regarded the 'feminine qualities' of nurses as appropriate to bedside care but as a profound hindrance to efficient administration, in that they encouraged concentration on minutiae at the expense of decisiveness. Salmon saw the direction forward as the promotion of a 'rational', 'masculine' style of management (Carpenter 1978). The masculinisation of the management of nurses has continued apace with the replacement of the Salmon system with a more generic managerial system following the Griffiths Report (Cousins 1988).

It can be seen that gender segregation correlates strongly with both inter- and intra-occupational differentials. The gender inequalities occurring in these two areas can be mutually reinforcing. The successful entry of a male minority into nursing, rather than diluting gender as a major defining factor in occupational differentiation, has exacerbated it by adding male managers to the nurse's burden of male doctors. Conversely, there is some evidence that the increasing entrance of women into medicine is leading to a degree of democratisation in the nurse-doctor relationship (Webster 1985).

Curing versus caring

One of the main themes emerging from the above discussion is that women's second class status both within and between the occupations of nursing and medicine is in part the result of assumptions founded upon a reductionist sociobiological model of gender role differentiation. According to such a model, women, as an extension of their maternal functions, possess expressive, emotional and caring qualities, while men are naturally more instrumental, rational, scientific and decisive. This social construction of the female role has been described by Hearn (1982) as the 'patriarchal feminine'; feminine because it accords to the feminine, 'caring' stereotype; patriarchal because in doing so it reinforces female subordination.

The patriarchal feminine is not simply a descriptive exercise, but involves judgement about the value of various human activities. Those activities which are categorised as being in the male domain are valued more highly than those adjudged appropriate for women (Sayers 1982). Nor is it simply a matter of adjudicating the merits of discrete tasks. Whole occupations are subject to differential rewards, according to whether they are categorised as 'men's' or 'women's' work (Crompton and Sanderson 1990).

The patriarchal feminine is not, however, the only interpretation open to those who accept 'given' gender differences. An alternative position attaches positive rather than negative evaluations to what are seen as immutable womanly traits. A number of radical feminists (for example, Firestone 1979 [1971]) posit biologistic explanations for the sexual division of labour, treating it as a natural, rather than socially generated division (Gamarnikow 1978).

However, other feminists take a more socialised view in explaining women's greater investment in caring and emotional labour. For example, Cline and Spender, in explaining why women place more emphasis on emotional aspects of their lives than men do, argue that:

> The overriding reason that women manipulate their emotions more than men is the fact that in general they have less independent access to money, power, authority or status in society. Their position as a subordinate group crucially determines the amount of time and energy they give to managing their emotions in order to build up men's egos. Because they lack other resources, women make a resource out of feeling (1987:120-121).

In consonance with the argument that emotional labour is subject to gender division, many nursing theorists accept the existence of a skills\caring, male\female dichotomy. This is hardly surprising, given that caring is seen as a core, and indeed unique, attribute of nursing. Defence of the importance of emotional labour is therefore central to the affirmation of nursing's worth (Robinson 1991). The battleground therefore becomes how the various attributes of nursing and medicine are to be evaluated:

> As long as fields that are stereotypically male, highly technological and illness orientated are held in higher esteem than those that have been stereotypically female, focusing on long-term care, quality of life and health maintenance, there is little reason to foresee major changes in interprofessional relationships (Webster 1985:317).

Claims for occupational equality are based on the assertion that female attributes are at least equal to male characteristics and that the 'feminine' tasks performed by nurses are of equal worth to the 'masculine' work of doctors (Gordon 1991). As Salvage puts it, 'Nurses/women should realise that doctors/men have much to learn from them' (1985:171). In essence, this strategy entails nursing theorists attempting to transform gender relations through an innovative attempt to emasculate the patriarchal feminine by turning it on its head.

Aims and method

Thus far I have examined how gender inequalities influence the institutional relations of medicine and nursing. However, this does not illustrate how these inequalities affect action at a clinical level, nor, indeed, how that action helps to maintain or transform structural inequalities. In line with critical realist concerns, my empirical enquiries were directed to the question of how the social structure of patriarchy influences social action and vice versa.

Much of the information presented here came from the intensive care unit. The number of subjects observed in the intensive care unit, disaggregated for occupation, sex and position, were as follows:

Table 6\1
Nursing and medical grades by sex

	Female	Male
Nurses		
Sister\Charge Nurse	4	0
Staff Nurse	28	3
Nursing Auxiliary	4	0
Total	36	3
Doctors		
Consultant	0	10
Registrar	1	3
Senior House Officer	5	5
Total	6	18

In addition to participant observation in the Intensive Care Unit, I used two other sources of empirical information. Firstly, I included questions about gender issues in the interviews with nurses from the Suburban Hospital. Secondly, I sought an independent empirical input. As a male nurse, I was very much involved in the social setting I was examining.[4] Given the crucial importance of gender to the topic I was addressing, I felt that techniques of empirical investigation which relied exclusively on my own sensibilities would be inadequate. As a consequence, I requested the collaboration of a female colleague who worked on a medical unit in the Metropolitan Hospital. Informing her of the problematics that I was considering, and the tentative conclusions that were emerging from my investigations, I asked her to record any nurse-doctor interactions, or statements by nurses or doctors that she felt were pertinent, either in support of my ideas, or in contradiction to them.[5]

A further technique that I used in this Chapter was formal quantification of some of the data. The purpose of this exercise was not to offer strong proofs for my claims. Rather, simple counting techniques were used to strengthen the evidence gained from qualitative techniques; to render explicit quantification that was already contained implicitly in the data I had gathered; and to give a general impression of the data, thus contextualising the extracts of interaction included in the chapter (Silverman 1985).

In order to tease out the significance of patriarchal relations to the occupational position of nurses, I focused enquiries on three questions:

1. How did gender permutations influence the nature of inter- and intra-occupational interaction?

2. Did female nurses utilise the concepts of patriarchy or gender in their understanding of their occupational position?

3. How did popular stereotyping of nurses' sexuality affect their occupational position?

Gender permutations and power

The effects of gender upon nurse-doctor interaction were measured by observing the interactions of four different combinations: female nurses and doctors; male nurses and doctors; male doctors and nurses; female doctors and nurses, and by studying the attitudes of female nurses to their gender roles.

Female and male nurses and doctors

The first thing I noted was that the gender of a nurse appeared to have little effect on their interaction with doctors. The male nurses studied were not observed to have any marked increase in authority in relation to doctors as compared to their female counterparts. In the formal occupational setting at least, the quality of interaction between male nurses and doctors and female nurses and doctors seemed very similar.[6]

Support for this contention came from counting the number of times male and female nurses were observed to make evaluative comments to doctors in reply to medical requests. While lack of comment by nurses does not necessarily reflect subservience in that silence can mean considered consent, the act of comment is indicative of assertiveness in that it entails an assumption by the nurse that her/his opinion is important.

It should be noted that I observed only three male nurses. All of them were junior staff nurses. It was therefore impossible to disaggregate the effects of their being in a junior position within the health care hierarchy from the effects of their gender. Their lowly status may have played an important part in the fact that they were no more assertive than female nurses. Nevertheless, if there were significant differences in interactions between male and female nurses and doctors, it might be assumed that these would be manifest even at junior levels.

Table 6\2

Occurrences of evaluative verbal responses by staff nurses in reply to doctors' clinical requests by sex of nurse

	Female %	Male %
Commented to doctor about request	28	22
Complied without comment	72	78
Base	53	36

$$[X^2 = 0.15; 1 \text{ d.f.}; p < 0.05].$$

The association between gender and likelihood of talking back to doctors was not statistically significant.

Female and male doctors and nurses

In contrast to the homogeneity of male and female nurses in their interactions with doctors, the interactions of female doctors with nurses were markedly different from some of their male colleagues. Two instances which occurred on the same day illustrate this point. The first involved a male senior house officer who was preparing to perform an aseptic procedure, and who was being assisted by a nurse. His sole verbal communication with the nurse during the entire episode consisted of the demand "Gloves!". At the end of the procedure he left the bedside without a word, leaving the nurse to clear up his debris.

The second involved a female SHO who was also performing an aseptic technique. As well as talking to the patient, the doctor also greeted the nurse, engaging in small talk with both nurse and patient throughout the procedure. Her requests were also expressed in a far more polite manner:

Transcript 6\1
Intensive Care Unit

SHO(F) Sorry, would you mind opening these gloves for me ... thanks.

On completing the procedure, she tidied away all her waste rather than leaving the nurse to do it.

This is not to say that all male doctors were as pompous as the one noted above. Indeed, there was considerable variation in the behaviour of male doctors towards nurses. Nor was it the case that there were no exceptions to the rule of sisterly love, as the following interaction between a staff nurse and a newly arrived doctor demonstrates:

Transcript 6\2
Metropolitan Hospital Medical Unit

SN(F)   Hello, I'm Forename, I staff here. You must be the new JHO.

SHO(F) Actually, Staff Nurse, I am Doctor Surname and I happen to be a senior house officer.

Nevertheless, it was generally true that most female doctors were considerably more egalitarian than most of their male counterparts.[7]

A quantitative indication of this came from counting the number of times doctors were prepared to tidy up after themselves, rather than leaving debris for nurses to dispose of. While 65% of female doctors observed cleaned up their clinical waste after procedures, the figure was only 36% for male doctors. Even when consultants, all of whom were male, and who were notably cavalier in their attitude towards procedures, were excluded from the equation, the difference remained statistically significant.

The individual variations in behaviour noted are a reminder that while gender may be an important factor in inter-occupational interaction, it is not the only one. Other aspects of status difference have considerable influence.

The fact that nurses' gender had far less impact on the quality of inter-occupational interaction than that of doctors probably indicates the power differential that exists between the two groups overall. Being in a weaker occupation means that nurses have less opportunity to engineer the quality of relationships. The inability of male nurses to utilise the advantages of their gender is the result of the ascription to nursing of a position of female subordination. The very factors that afford male nurses intra-occupational advantage work against them in inter-occupational power relations. Conversely, because of their position of authority, doctors have considerable latitude in deciding how they are going to interact with members of other occupations. They have the opportunity to avail themselves of the power that they implicitly possess if they wish to, or to act in a more egalitarian fashion if they do not.

These conclusions support Gamarnikow's (1978) thesis that patriarchal mechanisms segregate jobs, rather than individuals. Individuals entering jobs not associated with their sex find themselves in a contradictory position. Thus, ironically, female doctors can, if they wish, enjoy the patriarchal dominance over nursing that goes with their job, while, in their relations with doctors, male nurses share in the gendered subordination of their occupation.

Nurses' attitudes to gender issues

There was a militancy apparent in many nurses concerning doctors' assumptions about their inferior gender and occupational roles. Even when they acceded to performing 'handmaiden' activities, they often did so with bad grace, as the following incident demonstrates:

Transcript 6\3
Intensive Care Unit

The phone in the doctors' room rang. As all the doctors and nurses on duty were busy with other tasks and unavailable to answer it, a female staff nurse left her tea break to take the call. It was a message for a consultant who was on another phone at the time. The nurse spent several minutes standing in silence beside the consultant until he had finished his call and then informed him of the content of the other. She then returned to her tea and exclaimed to the other nurses on their break:

SN(F)   Nurse, cleaner, secretary, receptionist, that's all they think we are. The old sod didn't even say thank you!

Questioning about general attitudes to gender issues elicited ambiguous responses. A minority of ICU nurses (4 out of the 19 nurses specifically asked) expressed the view that occupational gender differences were to be explained by men having careers while women simply had jobs until they started a family. These differences in work experiences were seen as reflecting natural differences in the roles of the sexes. Nurses with these sorts of views tended to be meeker in their interactions with doctors. Others were considerably more assertive in their attitudes towards their gendered position.

SN(F)   I don't think being a women makes any difference to your ability to do a job of work. A woman can do this job or any other job just as well as a man. We're all the same under the skin.

This transcript indicates that not all nurses accepted the ascription of different faculties to women, preferring to express their feminism through the valorisation of a humanist universalism. However, others did see women as more caring.

Transcript 6\5
Medical Ward

SP   Do you think men and women bring different attributes to health care.

SN(F)   Hmmm, yes, I think so. I think women are more caring than a lot of men. I'm not saying that men don't do a good job, but they aren't as involved with their patients as women are. Maybe it's because some of us are mothers. Whatever, it's a real strength when you're caring for people with terrible problems.

SP   Do you think that that goes for male nurses?

SN(F)   Some of them, yea, but then again, some of them are more like women than women are [laughs].

The final comment here is an indication of structured inequality along the line of (perceived) sexual orientation. One way of dealing with men who enter female-dominated occupations is to denigrate them along homophobic lines, which enables them to be stripped of some of the structural advantages that would normally accrue to them because of their gender.

Criticising sexist individuals

Gender inequality was used by nurses on occasion to explain the authoritarianism of doctors, as the following exclamation of a ward nurse immediately after an altercation with a junior house officer demonstrates:

Transcript 6\6
Metropolitan Hospital Medical Unit

> SN(F): If that boy thinks we're little women here at his beck and call, he's going to have to learn the hard way. He's nothing but a wee male chauvinist pig!

Criticism like this was reserved for those male doctors who were openly bombastic. Sexism was seen as an individual attribute of specific doctors rather than an institutional ethos. Nurses tended not to accept that medical patriarchy was a generalised phenomenon. An example of the tendency to explain power differentials in functional terms was given by two Suburban Hospital nurses:

Transcript 6\7
Surgical Ward

> SP   Do you think the position of nurses relative to doctors has anything to do with the position of women in society in general?

> SN(F)   I haven't even thought about it.

> EN(F)   I don't know, to be honest. Because if you're talking about JHOs, it doesn't even come into consideration that they're men, you know. It doesn't for me, because they are so junior and they rely on us so much, you do feel more in control of them...

> SN(F)   And the more senior ones, well, they can tell us what to do because they're more senior, not because they're men.

However, the individualist explanations found in this study are certainly not shared by many nursing theorists. They may not even be entirely representative of clinical nurses' attitudes, as the published opinion of one student nurse demonstrates:

> So why do we nurses find ourselves in this [subservient] situation? Nursing is, and always has been, 'women's work' and medicine a man's world (Jones 1987:59).

Female nurses' attitudes to male nurses

Female nurses in this study were far more willing to ascribe general categorisations to male nurses. The success of senior male nurses was often put down to their sex. Male nurses in the clinical area, and therefore relatively junior in the nursing hierarchy, were invariably regarded as being on their way to higher things, once again because of their sex. My position as a former clinical nurse now working in a university meant that I did not escape the brunt of this perception. The perception of one nurse that my move from the clinical area into the educational sector was an example of a typically male career pattern was noted in Transcript 2\3. Similar attitudes were noted in other nurses, who were too polite to point the finger directly at me:

SP   What do you think people make of male nurses?

SN(F)   Well, I think sometimes they resent them a wee bit. When you see the likes of [male manager 1] or [male manager 2]. I mean, they just flew up into management, and from what I've heard, [male manager 1] was hopeless as a nurse. Why should they get promoted just because they're men? I mean, its not because they were brilliant on the wards.

SP   Why do you think they got promoted so fast?

SN(F)   I just think the management likes them. Maybe they think they'll stay around. I don't know, but, as I say, nine times out of ten, its certainly not because they're brilliant clinical nurses.

While their gender opened up greater career opportunities for male nurses, this did not mean that it gave clinical male nurses any advantage over their female counterparts in the immediate situation that they worked in. Barring an underlying resentment of female nurses about the unfairness of promotional opportunities for men, I found little difference in the attitudes and behaviour of other ICU nurses towards male and female ward nurses of the same grade.

However, another source of resentment of female nurses towards their male colleagues was expressed in interviews with Suburban Hospital nurses. This concerned the reputed indolence of many male nurses.

Transcript 6\9
Surgical Ward

SN(F)   I don't know how to say this, but male nurses are sometimes a bit slack. They tend not to be too fond of the hard work. Now, I'm not saying all of them are like that [laughs]. I'm sure you were an exception, but it's certainly noticeable that a good few of them are.

SP   Are they allowed to get away with it?

SN(F)   Well, it depends who's in charge, who's around. They wouldn't get away with it with me. I wouldn't be behind the door in telling them they were slacking if I thought I was having to do their work for them.

SP   Do you think male nurses are treated any differently?

SN(F)   If they do their work, then they're treated just the same as anybody. But someone that's slacking, whether they be a man or a women, can't really complain if them they're leaning on lets them know about it.

SP   So they don't get preferential treatment?

SN(F)   Och well, I suppose there's some that would dance around them, but there's a lot more would be suspicious of them. For the most part people just get on with the job, and don't pay too much attention to if its a man or a women you're doing it with, as long as they're pulling their weight.

My colleague in the Metropolitan Hospital Medical Unit found nurses even more willing to criticise male nurses for their laziness.

Transcript 6\10
Metropolitan Hospital Medical Unit

SRyan   Do you think male nurses are lazy?

EN(F)   Sure, you know they are. Some of them wouldn't know work if it hit them in the face.

SRyan   Do you think they are less caring?

EN(F)   Well now, to be fair to some of them, they're very good at psychological care. They're not afraid to sit on someone's bed and talk things out with them. But other types of care, well.

SRyan   How do you mean?

EN(F)   Well, to put it bluntly, even the best ones would rather run a mile than clean up shit.

The reason why male indolence and coprophobia was not such an issue in the intensive care unit could be related to the fact that each nurse on the unit was allocated to a single patient for the day, and was therefore obliged to carry out all areas of nursing care for that patient, whether they liked it or not. It could also be that my own gendered position coloured my observations.

Within the clinical focus of this study, the mechanisms by which men were able to advance themselves within nursing administration were not observed. This is significant, because it means that the generation of male hegemony within nursing management lies outside the doing of nursing. Examination of what these mechanisms are would be a fruitful point of departure for further research. The focus of that research would need to be those people located in health service administration, who have responsibilities for promotion.

The persuasiveness of credentialism

It may seem strange that while nurses viewed the position of their own job in terms of gender, they did not extend this outlook to their analysis of the position of medicine. After all, the positions of the two occupations are inextricably linked, and the brute fact of gender segregation appears to be obvious. However, the difference in attitude of female nurses to male nurses and to male doctors may be due to a difference in familiarity that they have about the processes of occupational advancement.

Because of a high degree of occupational segregation, nurses do not have a great deal of knowledge about how occupational advancement operates for doctors. They are confronted by doctors as people already possessing enabling qualifications and legal licence. These entitlements to occupational superiority are portrayed as resulting exclusively from a meritocratic process. It is hardly surprising, therefore, that nurses find it difficult to form a generalised gendered critique of the position of their medical counterparts.[8] This is testament to the justificatory power of credentialism in the maintenance of occupational closure (Berlant 1975).

Because nurses have had direct experience of the conditions pertaining in the processes of occupational advancement within their own occupation, they take a more cynical attitude towards them. Often either they, or someone they know, has been passed over in favour of a male colleague. This familiarity means that gender bias can less easily be hidden by the guise of functionalist justifications such as educational or experiential differentials.

While most nurses accepted that the position of doctors was largely due to the credentials they had accrued, this did not mean that they necessarily saw doctoring as a more important facet of health care than the activities that nurses were involved in. A number of nurses expressed their belief in the importance of nursing care in the promotion of health. The debate about the relative merits of technological intervention and human kindness was illustrated by a brief altercation between a junior doctor and a senior staff nurse, which resulted from the nurse expressing her incredulity that the doctor was capable of lifting someone off a commode.

JHO(M) Anyone can do a nurse's job, but there's not many people that can do what I can do.

SN(F) Oh yea? You wouldn't know how to care for your own granny if you had to. There's more to helping people than sticking needles in them, you know.

This interaction is interesting both because it indicates the positive evaluation many nurses put upon the caring role of nursing and as an example of the degree of assertiveness of nurses in their relationships with medical colleagues.

Sexual stereotyping

The final aspect of patriarchy I wish to deal with is the relationship between sexuality and power. The ideological basis for power divisions predicated upon sexuality lies in this instance in the sexual stereotyping of nurses. This entails the image of them as being sexually permissive, most notably with young male doctors. By portraying nurses as sexual objects, these stereotypes provide further ideological support for the dominance of male doctors in the sexual division of labour.

This ideology has a wider import than its effect on nurse-doctor power relations. It reflects a more generalised attempt to place women in a subservient position. Muff (1982) has argued that the sexual stereotypes that nurses are subjected to are the result of myths generated by a male fear of the feminine other.

It is easy to see the relationship between the mythologies and stereotypes of women and those of nurses. Their purposes are the same: to provide easy solutions to the complexities of human relationships, to obviate the need for men to understand each women (nurse) as an individual by providing categories within which to 'file' her, and to transform the woman (nurse) into *his* ideal to make her more acceptable and accessible and to lessen his guilt by association. Stereotypes are seductive. Once their use becomes habitual (and it has), the conformity of women becomes imperative. No longer merely defence mechanisms or shortcuts for the lazy, these stereotypes are standards by which all women (nurses) are measured and thus are tools of oppression (1982:120-121).

While Muff's psychoanalytic approach demonstrates the crucial significance of this ideology, it tends towards an ahistorical and immutable conception of mythical stereotypes. Kalisch and Kalisch (1982b; 1982c and 1982d) have argued that this particular portrayal of nurses is an historically recent phenomenon. Up until the 1960s, media portrayal of nurses was largely that of chaste young women. During the era of sexual 'liberation' this altered radically, with nurses being increasingly portrayed as promiscuous playthings of their medical colleagues.

Kalisch and Kalisch do not speculate as to why this may be so. However, if it is accepted that the images of nurses reflect the images of women in general, a pattern can be identified. Sexual liberalisation was a double-edged sword. While it allowed for greater personal freedom, it also brought into starker relief the subordination of women through their sexual roles. If male power and supremacy is expressed through sexuality (Millett 1971), then openness about sex will exacerbate its significance for male domination. In eras when sex is repressed, the domestic, caring roles of women are more prominent aspects of justificatory ideologies for their oppression. Thus the image of nurses prior to the 1960s was often one of altruistic angels (Kalisch and Kalisch 1982b; 1982c and 1982d).

Because of the nature of their work, which involves intimate contact with bodies, and indeed with unpleasant bodily functions and dysfunctions, nurses seem to be singled out more than most female occupational groups as the butt of sexual stereotyping. The fear of the other is exacerbated by the other's intrusion into physical aspects of life which are normally closely guarded secrets. Consequently, the mythical stereotypes employed are all the more grotesque. Nurses' intrusions into the bodies of others are countered by the demeaning of nurses' own bodies.

Despite the ubiquity of images in popular culture which portray nurses as the sexual chattels of their medical colleagues, I found no empirical evidence to suggest that the hospital units studied were simmering fleshpots whose primary purpose was to facilitate the libidinous proclivities of young doctors. No evidence of intimate relationships between doctors and nurses in the ICU was discovered, although it has to be admitted that by their very nature such interactions would tend to be discreetly handled by those involved. Analysis of the company nurses reported keeping on evenings out showed that the people they socialised with were rarely medical personnel. Indeed, only twice did nurses inform me that they had been in the company of doctors, and even then it had been in the context of group outings. While it would be overstating the case to say that intimate contacts between male doctors and female nurses never occur, it does seem that the myths about nurse's sexual behaviour are exactly that - myths.

It is hardly surprising that nurses find this state of affairs particularly galling. The level of their resentment was displayed in a discussion about a grossly sexist portrayal of nurses in a daily newspaper. The conversation was concluded with the following comment on the writer of the piece by a young staff nurse:

Transcript 6\12
Intensive Care Unit

SN(F)   I just wish that one day that bastard becomes sick and I get to nurse
        him. I tell you, he'll never have another sexual thought in his life by
        the time I've finished with him.

The attitude of nurses such as the one cited above is significant, as it demonstrates that nurses are not prepared to accept such an oppressive and reductive ideological construct of their nature. In addition, the vociferousness with which rejection of this stereotype was expressed indicates that sexual stereotypical utterances, if they were made in the presence of nurses, would receive short shrift. Indeed, the fact that stereotypical expressions were absent from the 'frontstage' discourse of male doctors in the ICU shows the effectiveness of nurses' rejection.

However, backstage talk of male doctors amongst themselves is another matter entirely. As a temporarily employed nurse, my access during this research to the informal medical milieu was limited. However, during my nursing career, I was, on occasion, privy to all-male backstage conversations which involved the usage of sexual stereotypes by male doctors about female nurses.[9] That this sort of attitude is still prevalent within medical culture was indicated by an article written by a doctor the *Nursing Times*, in which he recounted the punch line in a medical student review that he had attended: 'Nurses. Great shag, thick as pigshit' (Hammond 1994:52).

If it is taken that it remains the case that sexist stereotypes are embedded in male medical culture, then the success of nurses preventing them being realised in public discourse is of limited effect, in that stereotypes still animate doctors' attitudes to their nursing colleagues, even though they do not openly express them.

Sexual harassment

Sexuality, as a factor in patriarchal relations, is not limited to ideological denigration. Game and Pringle (1984) argue that sexual ideology can be used as a basis for actions that repress women in a more direct manner, namely sexual harassment. Therefore, a full examination of the relationship between sexuality and inter-occupational relations requires investigation of the issue of physical oppression of female nurses by male doctors.

Game and Pringle note that 'Doctors exercise not only the power of the father but direct sexual power over nurses. Medical dominance is reaffirmed by sexual domination' (1984:108). They noted that surgeons in operating theatres, especially, had the power to enforce sexual contact on nurses as part of their nursing duties, illustrating their point with the following transcript of a theatre nurse's statement.

> For a start you're all running around in things like pyjamas. There are expanses of exposed thighs. Doctors hitch their jockettes up over their hipbone ... the surgeon will say 'nurse, I've got an itchy thigh' - and of course they're gowned and gloved and you have to go and scratch them - or wipe their brow when there's no sweat ... It's so grossly humiliating but you *can't* refuse to do it (1984:108-109, emphasis in original).

I found little evidence of this sort of behaviour in the intensive care unit. This is not as contradictory as it might first seem. As Game and Pringle point out, there are significant exceptions to this pattern of sexual domination. They point to two circumstances which have the effect of reducing the possibility of harassment. They argue that in specialist units where nurses are highly skilled and knowledgeable, and in units where there is a significant proportion of female doctors, male doctors will be restrained from sexual harassment. Both of these circumstances pertained in the ICU.

Unfortunately, it would seem that interactions in the ICU may be the exception rather than the rule. Evidence from the Metropolitan Hospital Medical Unit demonstrates that sexual harassment remains a fairly common experience for nurses. One consultant was infamous for approaching every new nurse who started to work on the ward, looking for an engagement or marriage ring, and if discovering both to be absent, asking the nurse what sort of underwear she wore. Nurses' reaction to this kind of harassment varied considerably. The response of one nurse gained immortality amongst her colleagues. She grabbed the consultant, pushed him into a room, and demanded, given that he was making such a big deal about sex, that he show her what he had to offer. She was never troubled by him again. Unfortunately, for many nurses, this sort of a response was not an option, and they were forced to suffer indignity in embarrassed silence.

Evidence from the nurses in the Suburban Hospital reinforces the impression that sexual harassment by some doctors remains commonplace.

Transcript 6\13
Medical Ward

SP   Have you ever been sexually harassed?

SN(F)   Well, nothing really bad, but of course you do get the smarmy ones who are for ever putting their arms around you or pawing you. I find the cold shoulder usually works, but some of them can be persistent.

SP   What do you feel about doctors that harass?

SN(F)   Well, you can't respect them very much. What they are doing is totally unprofessional. They are just abusing their position.

From the evidence gathered, I think it fair to concur with Game and Pringle that sexual harassment remains an important factor in gendered relations within health care, but that its incidence will vary greatly according to situational factors. However, I think that the nurse's second reply in the above transcription prompts an important qualification to their thesis that sexual power reinforces occupational power. Rather than using sexual harassment to enhance their occupational power, those doctors that indulged in it seemed to be using their occupational power to enable them to get away with harassment. By using their power in this way, they actually forfeited their moral authority and some of their professional status.

Sexual behaviour was not entirely absent from the ICU. Occasional instances of sexual innuendo and mild flirtation were noted. However, it appeared that these

115

were indulged in voluntarily by both males and females. Evidence that nurses did not feel coerced into these sorts of came from the following interaction between myself and an ICU staff nurse.

> *Transcript 6\14*
> *Intensive Care Unit*

> SP   Do you think that any sexual harassment goes on here?

> SN(F) Hah! They wouldn't dare. No, seriously, no one down here has pushed it too far with me. I suppose some of them think they're God's gift, but no one pays a blind bit of notice to them.

> SP   But you do hear quite risqué conversations.

> SN(F) Oh, for God's sake, that's only fun. It's just people having a bit of *craic*[10] and enjoying themselves. You shouldn't read too much into that sort of thing.

Given that nurses reciprocated in these mild sexual interactions, and indeed sometimes initiated them, it would seem that such interactions fall well outside the ambit of sexual harassment, if we define sexual harassment as 'non-reciprocal, unsolicited, (usually) masculine behaviour which asserts (usually) a girl's or woman's sexual identity over her identity as a person' (Farley 1978:14). Indeed, it could be argued that his type of interaction between young heterosexuals of the opposite sex who work in close proximity is entirely unremarkable. However, we should keep in mind that identification of the demarcation line between sexual joking and sexual harassment is highly problematic (Halson 1991). Moreover, while this sort of behaviour may not be sexual harassment, a case could be made that it has significant unintended consequences,[11] in that it highlights gender differentiation, and thus reinforces medical power by underlining the sexual division of labour.

The influence of lateral 'female' roles[12]

Paradoxically, given that fixation with the sexuality of nurses appears to be a relatively recent media phenomenon, it appears that the dearth of romantic involvement between doctors and nurses that now pertains was not always the case. A significant proportion of senior doctors in the ICU and Metropolitan Hospital Medical Unit were married to nurses or former nurses. The lack of interest shown by younger doctors in their nursing colleagues as prospective partners may be partially the result of the large influx of women into medicine. With the progressive equalising of the gender ratio, male doctors have an increasing opportunity to develop personal relationships with their peers. A number of doctor-doctor personal relationships were noted in the study.

There also seems to be a change in the way nurses view the prospect of doctors as future partners. Earlier studies of nursing almost universally identified an ambivalence on the part of nurses towards their occupation (Davis and Oleson 1963; Dingwall 1977; Simpson 1979; Weitzman 1982). These writers, whose ideological bent ranges from interactionism and phenomenology to functionalism and feminism, all seem to agree that the occupational commitment of nurses was compromised by lateral female roles and the prospect of family life and motherhood. If nurses gave their private ambitions precedence over their career aspirations, then seeking a high status partner from the medical profession would seem a feasible tactic.

Contrary to the conclusions of previous studies, which posited that, because of their gender, nurses rarely regarded their employment as a career, I would argue that for many nurses this is no longer the case. While I have already noted that a minority of nurses in the ICU continued to regard their work as an interval before the adoption of the domestic role, most were quite definite that they were in the occupation for reasons to do with the occupation itself, whether this was simply to earn a wage, or because of the satisfaction that being in a 'caring profession' brings. Moreover, a number of nurses in the ICU (9 out of the 19 with whom it was discussed) explicitly stated that, notwithstanding their desire to marry, they saw their job as a career which they expected to follow throughout their working lives.

Male doctors' attentions towards female doctors rather than nurses caused amusement rather than resentment in the female nurses observed. This was evidenced by nurses' reactions to several emotional imbroglios between female and male doctors which occurred on the Metropolitan Hospital Medical Unit where more junior medical personnel worked. Their attitude was summed up by one rather cynical staff nurse:

Transcript 6\15
Metropolitan Hospital Medical Unit

SN(F)   It's great fun watching them break each others' hearts!

With the increasing perception of nursing as a career in itself, the instrumental motivation of using it to find a marriage partner has become, if not completely defunct, at least increasingly anachronistic. Of course, the difficulties that nurses face in developing their careers should not be underestimated, in that the organisational structures in which they work remain oriented to the traditional male career path which assumes that uninterrupted, full-time employment is the standard. Women's employment patterns, often characterised by career breaks and part-time working is regarded an aberration from the norm. This 'manpower' thinking results in a profound devaluation of female nurses within the health care labour market (Davies 1995).

Conclusion: two steps forward and one step back

In conclusion, it can be seen that gender remains one of the most important factors in nurses' experience. Its effect, however, does appear to be changing over time. I would contend that these changes reflect general trends in the position of women in our society. If the subordination of nurses in the Nightingale era was an extension of the overtly oppressed situation that women found themselves in at that time, the rather more convoluted and mutable nature of nurses' relations with doctors that pertain today reflect the gradual alteration of the position of women as a whole. We should be cautious, however, about seeing this process as a uniform, if exceedingly gradual, march towards gender equality.

Certainly, there were a number of aspects identified in this study that indicated that change was taking place in this direction. Most notable of these was the refusal of many nurses to acquiesce without objection to the subordinate position that some doctors expected them to take. These actions were predicated upon an increasingly positive self-evaluation of nurses about their role as female workers. This self-evaluation was also evidenced in their rejection of stereotypical images which denigrated their sexuality. In addition, the increasing proportion of female doctors seems to be leading to an attenuation of patriarchy in nurse-doctor power relations. These factors bear testament to the claim that social institutions are not reified entities, beyond the grasp of the actors that live within them, but are constantly either maintained or transformed by social agency (Bhaskar 1989a; Giddens 1984). Women, as both nurses and doctors, have been able to partially transform their occupational position within health care institutions. While the transformation of patriarchal structures into more equitable gender relations may be far from complete, as the continuing practice of sexual harassment illustrates, the historical evidence cited in Chapter Three indicates that the degree of progress should not be underestimated.

However, unfounded optimism should be guarded against. In examining the trajectory of patriarchal structures over time, the increase in male managerial authority over the last quarter of a century must be taken into account. While female nurses are certainly aware of this process, to date little has been done to tackle it. Indeed, the indications are that nursing will increasingly become an occupation divided between male managers and female ward workers. Following the Griffiths report (1983) into NHS management, the Salmon system has been abandoned, with lines of authority exclusive to nurses being replaced by a flexible, generic system of management. One of the effects of the Griffiths reforms is that nurse managers now have to compete for their positions with managers from predominantly male occupations such as medicine and private business. That this has exacerbated gender inequalities in health care management is indicated by the fact that only 3% of the district general management posts that were created by the reforms were filled by women (Cousins 1988). Nor should this be seen as merely a matter of the gender of individuals who fill these positions of power. We also need to take account of the overwhelmingly masculine *culture* of health service management - a culture that does not fully take account of women's lives and careers and which, as a result, disadvantages female nurses on grounds of their gender (Davies 1995).

There is bitter irony in the fact that at a time when the problems of gender in relation to doctors are being at least partially resolved, the issue has reappeared with just as much vigour in a different locus.

Notes

1. As I noted in Chapter One, this triad of structures omits an extremely important structural mechanism within Irish society - that of sectarianism. While this book is limited to discussion of factors that have a more general pertinence, this does not obviate the fact that much work needs to be done in theorising how sectarianism in Irish society affects the working lives of groups such as nurses.
2. This concept of subservience certainly remained in the eyes of many sociological commentators. A good example of the nurse being regarded as unproblematically subordinate can be found in Freidson's (1970) description of the position of 'paramedical' occupations.
3. Gamarnikow makes the important point that categorising occupations along gender lines is not simply an arithmetic exercise:

> The sexual division of labour ... situates individuals in jobs and designates jobs as sex specific. This is an ideological operation specific to patriarchy. It is not an *ex post facto* description of occupational sex ratios. Thus it is possible for some women to enter 'male' jobs and vice versa without these jobs losing ideological designation as sex specific: rather, this becomes an individualised act, frequently resulting in contradictory and difficult work relations (1978:101).

4. This is one of the most important points of anti-positivist sociology. It is expressed clearly (albeit in a sexist manner) by Elias:

> social as distinct from natural sciences are concerned with conjunctions of persons. Here, in one form or another, men face themselves; the 'objects' are also 'subjects'. The task of social scientists is to explore, and to make men understand, the patterns they form together ... The investigators themselves form part of these patterns. They cannot help experiencing them, directly or by identification, as immediate participants from within (1956:228).

Bhaskar accepts this qualification to the possibility of naturalism in the social sciences, noting that:

> social sciences are part of their own field of enquiry, in principle susceptible to explanation in terms of the concepts and laws of the

explanatory theories they employ; so that they are *internal* with respect to their subject matter in a way in which natural science is not (1989b:84).

However, Bhaskar views this 'limitation' less as an epistemological problem than as a praxical boon, in that it allows social science to play a part in the transformation of society. It will be remembered that I discussed this issue of the relationship of social science and its subject matter *vis-à-vis* sociology and nursing in Chapter Four.

5. I would like to record my thanks at this point to Sandra Ryan for her significant contribution to my research into the issue of gender.

6. previous research into this issue is rather ambiguous. While Benokraitis and Feagin (1986) and Game and Pringle (1984) have argued that male doctors interact with male nurses in a preferential manner, Mackay (1989) found little evidence that this was the case.

7. Once again, evidence from the literature on the relationship between female doctors and nurses is contradictory. Game and Pringle (1984) found that female doctors were more authoritarian than their male counterparts. The reason Game and Pringle gave for this was that, in order to keep up with the men, women doctors had to work hard to assert their position and could not afford to fraternise with nurses. On the other hand, nurses in Mackay's study tended to see female doctors as more approachable than male doctors.

8. This facet of social interaction reminds us of Bhaskar's observation that while society is a skilled accomplishment of active agents, 'the social world may be opaque to the social agents upon whose activity it depends' (1989b:4). One of the aspects of this opacity is the existence of what he calls 'unacknowledged conditions'. It would seem that the role gender plays in the occupational superordination of medicine is at least partially unacknowledged by nurses.

9. It should be noted that such backstage talk, involving males of both occupations, indicates that while there may be little difference in formal interactions between male doctors and male and female nurses, does not falsify Game and Pringle's (1984) thesis that male doctors treat male nurses as men first and nurses second. The reasons why these attitudes were not manifest frontstage in the ICU may involve the power of professional etiquette, which would tend to devalue such discourse as boorish. This is not to say that professionalism unproblematically countervails against sexism; in many ways the culture of professionalism, with its orientation to control and mastery, is inherently masculine (Davies 1995). However, aspects of professional ideology, such as the valorisation of affective neutrality, tend to preclude open expression of derogatory personalised discourse. I will discuss the capacity of professional ideology to inhibit the realisation of oppressive structural mechanisms more fully in the next chapter.

10. *Craic* is an Irish word that can be roughly translated as 'fun'.

11. Unintended consequences of social actions are another way in which the social world is obscured to individuals (Bhaskar 1989b). The social significance of unintended consequences was first recognised by Merton (1968 [1949]), who

argued that individual actions often contain latent functions of which the actor is unaware, but which serve to maintain the social institutions to which the actor belongs. Thus apparently irrational individual activities may contain a latent rationality at the level of social system. Giddens (1984) is equally convinced of the importance of unintended consequences in the reproduction of institutionalised practices. However, he rejects the functionalist aspect of Merton's argument on the grounds that it makes the unwarranted imputation that social systems have motivations, independent of the motivations of actors within them. Wielding Occam's razor, Giddens provides a more parsimonious explanation of unintended consequences:

> To understand what is going on no explanatory variables are needed other than those which explain why individuals are motivated to engage in regularized social practices across space and time, and what consequences ensue (1984:14).

In the case examined here, the motivations of the actors can be explained in terms of interactive pleasure, while the unintended consequence that ensues is the reinforcement of gender-based divisions of labour.

12. The concept of lateral roles was developed by Oleson and Whittaker (1968), who used it to denote processes of socialisation that occur outside the occupational setting, but which impinge upon occupational acculturation. They argued that for women, the most significant lateral role relates to expectations about their involvement in personal relationships and domestic labour.

7 Racism

Introduction

One of the most powerful critiques that mainstream feminism was subjected to in the 1980's emanated from black feminists, who argued that the examination of gender issues was inadequate, and indeed imperialist, if it ignored the issues of ethnicity and racism (Amos and Parmar 1984). The importance of ethnic inequality for the analysis of gender relations lies in the fact that the structure of racism will affect the form that patriarchy takes (Walby 1986).

Studies on the structural interpolations of patriarchy and racism tend to concentrate on the experiences of black or Asian women (for example, Parmar 1982; Phizacklea 1988). One of the primary aims of these studies is to demonstrate that the female experience of patriarchy is not a uniform one - that the racialised position of black and Asian women qualitatively alters their position in gender relations. In such circumstances, racism is seen as overdetermining patriarchally generated oppression.

The social situation being examined in this study is exceptional (at least as far as the literature is concerned) in that the structural mechanism of racism in this particular instance tended to attenuate, rather than reinforce the effects of patriarchy. This dichotomy resulted from the composition of the particular workforce under examination. In this case, the vast majority of health care workers belonging to racialised groups were doctors.[1] All of the nurses observed in the ICU and interviewed in the Suburban Hospital were white.

Given such a scenario, it might be expected that 'race' would be a significant status-determining characteristic. However, this was not the case; individuals who belonged to racialised groups were to a considerable extent shielded from the full brunt of racism.

The aim of this chapter is to examine the effects of racism upon relations between nurses and doctors, using Bhaskar's critical realism and Bourdieu's theory of practice as explanatory tools. However, before doing this, it is necessary to demonstrate that it is valid to describe racism in structural terms, and to discuss how structural racism articulates with racist attitudes and behaviour.

The two core features of social structures, according to critical realism (Craib 1984), are that they are *relational* (they involve enduring relations between the societal positions of actors) and that they possess *ontological depth* (their existence lies behind, and affects, manifest phenomena).

Racism certainly involves enduring relationships between agents in different social positions. Being black in a racist society entails being categorised in numerous ways that result in disadvantage. Racist engendered positions predate any of the individual actors now situated within them, and may well outlast them, albeit in modified forms. Moreover, *mutatis mutandis*, it is experienced by people in diverse social situations (including that of Ireland (McVeigh 1992)).[2]

This persistence over time and space also indicates ontological depth. Beneath manifestations of racism is an underlying set of social relationships. Racist acts cannot be adequately explained solely through elucidation of the attitudes of the individuals involved. Rex (1970) observes that such an approach, because it fails to address the origins of individual attitudes, leads to their reification. In order to avoid this static conception of racism, the articulation between racist acts, racist attitudes, and structural racism needs to be considered.

The first thing to note is that their relations are not invariant. Because social phenomena occur in open systems, social and psychological 'laws' can only be analysed as tendencies (Bhaskar 1989b). The attitudes and actions of individuals are not predetermined by the social structures within which they live. Rather, the practices they engage in will be influenced by the social position which they occupy - social position provides the means, media, rules and resources available to enable or coerce action (Bhaskar 1989a). Thus, individuals will enjoy more or less powerful and enabling positions in a society which displays structural racism, depending how they are categorised in racist terms. However, this does not mean that because people live in a racist society, they will necessarily display racist behaviour, or even possess racist attitudes. Nonetheless, there is pressure on them to do so, especially if they reside in the empowered camp of a racist divide, in that racist attitudes can provide an ideological rationalisation for the structural inequalities from which they may benefit.

The links between the ideology and practice of racism are even closer than this. Indeed, it should be noted that racism is entirely premised upon an ideological category, 'race' being nothing more than a reified social construction (Miles 1982). This does not mean, however, that it can be reduced to the status of superstructural epiphenomenon. Racism, although founded upon ideological assumptions which have little bearing to reality, nevertheless has real effects upon social relations.

In his portrayal of the relationship between material activity and ideology, Bhaskar attempts to avoid the twin errors of idealism and material reductionism. Rather than viewing ideas and actions as separate entities, he argues that 'all activity ... necessarily has an ideational component, that is to say that it is unthinkable except in so far as the agent has a conception of what s\he is doing and why s\he is doing it (in which of course s\he may be mistaken)' (Bhaskar 1989b:66). The parenthetic qualification is an important one in that it allows for the possibility of unintentional racism. Because the social world may be opaque to the actors within it, it is possible for actions to have the effect of maintaining racist structures without actors realising that they are doing so. Nevertheless, if we allow that individuals often act with reflexive intentionality, we must assume that there is frequently a connection between racist acts and racist ideas.

There is, however, another qualification that requires to be made in relation to the connection between thought and action - the possession of racist beliefs does not necessarily entail the performance of racist acts. By dint of the fact that the human psyche is an open system, attitudes should be regarded as tendencies, rather than iron determinants. To this end, it will be my contention that racism will usually only be manifested in circumstances which actors possessing racist attitudes regard as auspicious for its display.

In sum, racism is a structural phenomenon, displaying both relational power and ontological depth. Its effect upon action, however, cannot be construed in terms of constant conjunction. Rather, the relationship between structure and action can better be described as generative - with the former providing the conditions for the latter. Conversely, structural racism is dependent upon the consciousness and motivated action of agents, because it is that consciousness and action which maintains or transforms it.

Method

Almost all of the empirical data in this chapter comes from participant observation of nurses and doctors in the intensive care unit. The number of subjects observed in the ICU were: 39 nurses, all of whom were white Irish; and 24 doctors, five of whom belonged to racialised groups. The hypotheses I commenced with were:

1. The structural phenomenon of racism would to some degree inform relationships between white health workers and those belonging to racialised groups.

2. The occupational situation would affect the way in which racism was expressed.

'Race' and power

David Hughes's (1988), in an ethnographic study of nurse-doctor interaction in a British casualty unit, noted that a significant variable affecting the nurse-doctor relationship was the geographical origin of the doctor. Many of the doctors he studied were recent immigrants to Britain from the Asian sub-continent. Interactions with these doctors frequently involved a breakdown of nurses' deference.

Such was not the case in my study. The interaction of nurses with black or Asian doctors elicited little observed alteration in the balance of power. Indeed, the doctor in the unit most respected for his clinical knowledge was African. With a background in medical research which had furnished him with an impressive fund of information, he was frequently quizzed by nurses on the more esoteric aspects of the medical corpus. It was noticeable, however, that he made conspicuous efforts to ensure that his superior grasp of formal occupational knowledge was recognised. An example of this self-assertive strategy involved a demonstration of the diagnostic limitations of nurses. Much to his own amusement, the doctor asked in turn every nurse present in the unit to try to interpret a patient's chest X-ray. After several had failed to grasp the import of the image they were examining, he even provided a clue that the patient had suffered from tuberculosis about fifty years previously. To the evident satisfaction of their interrogator, not one nurse noticed that the patient had had half a lung removed! To my eternal shame, I was one of those tested.

That episodes such as this were part of a deliberate strategy, rather than an unselfconscious display of clinical knowledge, can be inferred from the following fieldnotes of a conversation between myself and this doctor.

Transcript 7\1
Intensive Care Unit

> I asked him what it was like coming to work in a place like this. He went over some of the pros and cons of his move ... [One con he identified was] that every time he got a new post, he had to start all over again. People automatically assumed that because he 'wasn't from here' he wouldn't know anything. Every time, he had to go through the same old routine before they accepted that he was good at his job. He wryly concluded: 'but I think people soon get the message'.

Another strategy adopted by some doctors from ethnic minorities was the utilisation of formal occupational power. For example, one Asian consultant was noted for his authoritarian manner. His attitude was normally one of distant superiority. He rarely talked to his nursing colleagues, and made little attempt to involve them in decision-making processes about patient care. When he did communicate with nurses, it was almost exclusively to gain information upon which to base his own decisions. Indeed, if he could get the information he needed from clinical records, he eschewed even this mode of interaction. Once he had made a decision, he rarely felt it necessary to explain the rationale behind it, as the following transcript of my observations illustrates:

Transcript 7\2
Intensive Care Unit

A male consultant arrives at the bedside with a female sister, during his morning round. He spends some minutes examining the charts detailing the patient's vital signs and the medication being given. He then lifts the blankets from the bottom of the bed and feels the pedal pulses of the unconscious patient. After this, he turns around, and moves off to wash his hands, without replacing the bedclothes or, apart from a vague Mmm, communicating with either the sister or the staff nurse looking after the patient. The implicit message in his silence is taken by the nurses to mean that he recommends no change in the patient's treatment. The staff nurse says nothing to him, though the sister begins to talk with him at the next bed (whether about the previous patient or not is impossible to tell). While she fixes the bedclothes, the staff nurses mutters under her breath. While her utterances are audible to the consultant, they are indecipherable. He gives no indication of hearing her.

The consultant's demeanour was not simply one of social distance. He was prepared to exercise his occupational authority in more direct ways. He did not balk at demonstrating his power to the point of chastising nurses in front of their patients, as the following fieldnote demonstrates:

Transcript 7\3
Intensive Care Unit

In the process of a 'ward round', the consultant comes across a heavily stained dressing.

CON(M)Who is looking after this patient?

SN(F)   I am.

CON(M)This is a disgrace. This dressing should have been changed hours ago.

(The staff nurse reddens, but does not reply)

SR(F)   The wound's being giving us a lot of trouble. There's a lot of exudate and we're having to replace the padding almost continually.

CON(M)Mmm. Is he pyrexial?'

This authoritarianism was rarely openly challenged by nurses. Overt demonstrations of dissatisfaction were restricted to some nurses withholding help or information from the consultant unless and until he specifically asked them. This exacerbated communication problems and increased mutual resentment (to say

126

nothing of the effect it had upon clinical efficiency). Nevertheless, interactions between nurses and this doctor displayed an aura of starched propriety, where nurses gave the outward appearance of 'knowing their place' in the occupational hierarchy.

The reality of racism

One possible explanation for the deference found in my study, in contrast to Hughes's (1988), is that racism is absent from Irish society. Such a hypothesis was, however, belied by the private complainings of nurses amongst themselves which indicated that the conceptions of 'race' and racial inferiority were utilised by at least some of them (*cf.* McVeigh 1992) . When nurses were on their own, or 'backstage' to use Goffman's (1969) term, professional propriety was dispensed with. During tea and meal breaks, and on other occasions when they were out of earshot of both doctors and patients, nurses often complained about what they regarded as unfair behaviour on the part of some of their medical colleagues. These complaints served as 'secondary adjustments' (Goffman 1968), allowing nurses to temporarily shed institutional assumptions about how they should think and behave. On occasion, they were expressed in racist terms:[3]

> *Transcript 7\4*
> *Intensive Care Unit*

> SN(F)   Who does he think he is, coming over here from the arse end of the world and telling us who were born and reared here what to do?

Racism was frequently elided with gender issues, as can be seen in a nurse's reaction to the consultant's behaviour recorded in Transcript 7\3:

> *Transcript 7\5*
> *Intensive Care Unit*

> SN(M)   Jesus, [Surname] was a really nasty to you on the round.

> SN(F)1 Yea, but at least [Sister] stood up for me.

> SN(F)2 Its out of order, treating us like that. They may treat women like skivvies in Pakistan, but I don't see why he should get away with it here.

We can see here an instance of how the articulation of structural mechanisms are manifest in interaction. The nurse is using racism as a means to devalue the patriarchal power of the doctor. We can also observe the hierarchy of structures pertaining in this situation. The fact that the doctor can exercise patriarchy openly with impunity, while the nurse can only use racism as a backstage secondary adjustment demonstrates the overriding significance of patriarchy.

Another point to be made about this transcript is the ambiguity of the remark about the treatment of women in Pakistan. It could be interpreted simply as a derogatory remark about the oppressive cultural *mores* of Pakistani society, rather than as an explicitly racist attack. However, I would argue that even if it were possible to distinguish between these two forms of criticism (and I am not convinced that it is), in this social situation such a distinction is not appropriate. Support for my contention comes from a transcript of a conversation that I had later with the same nurse on a similar topic.

Transcript 7\6
Intensive Care Unit

SN(F) They're [Asian men] all like that - spoiled rotten, every one of them. They just think they can do what they like and everyone should run after them.

SP That's a bit of a racist generalisation, isn't it?

SN(F) It isn't racist at all, it's a fact. If Pakis are like that, it isn't my fault, that they're arrogant b's (laughs).

In this conversation, in order to justify her statements about colleagues, the staff nurse uses the argument that it is possible to differentiate between objective, generalised critiques of groups and unsubstantiated racist slurs. However, by her use of the racist term 'Paki' in conjunction with the derogatory epithet 'arrogant b's', she succeeds in disproving her own argument.

I heard the term 'Paki' used on several occasions. However, it was the only explicitly racist name that I did hear. Racism was usually expressed more subtly. Nevertheless, despite their avoidance of grossly racist terms, a number of statements made by nurses could still be clearly described as racist. Take, for example, the following encounter, which continues the theme of medical arrogance:

Transcript 7\7
Intensive Care Unit

SN(F) Why is that man so bloody obnoxious?

SR(F) (Laughing) He can't help it. It's the way he's made. I'm afraid Pakistanis are like that.

The Sister's statement falls firmly within the parameters of Schermerhorn's description of racism as:

an ideology that sees an invariable connection between cultural behaviour and physical type. Hence it defines specific outgroups as having characteristic traits (usually detestable or in some way inferior) that are inherent outgrowths of their biological constructions (1970: 102)

While racist remarks frequently took the form of responses to doctors' arrogance, backstage racism was not limited to pathologised reactions to heavy-handed authoritarianism. More egalitarian doctors were also subject to prejudice:

Transcript 7\8
Intensive Care Unit

A staff nurse opens the door to enter a clinical room where she discovers a Palestinian doctor at prayer. After mumbling polite apologies, she retreats from the room. However, almost immediately the following interaction occurs.

SN(F)   That bloody Arab is praying again in the treatment room. How am I supposed to get my work done?

DOM(F) Huh, if he wants to go down on his hands and knees every ten minutes, you'd think he'd stay in his own country and do it.

SN(F)   Arabs!

She moves off shaking her head.

Even the African clinical expert was not totally immune, although racist remarks that referred to him tended to be patronising, rather than adversarial:

Transcript 7\9
Intensive Care Unit

SN(F) He's the smartest black person I've ever met.

Moreover, with the exception of the clinical expert, the relationship of white nurses and black doctors was considerably cooler and more formal than between white nurses and white doctors, irrespective of whether the nurses characterised the doctors as authoritarian.

However, this undercurrent of racism in the attitudes of some of the nurses did little to undermine the authority of the doctors concerned in face-to-face interactions. This is not to say that nurses were unproblematically subservient (we have already seen in Chapter Five that they were not), rather that the negotiating tactics that they used did not differ qualitatively to those they used with white doctors. Specifically, I saw no evidence of the types of interactions that were noted in Hughes' (1988) study: nurses in my study were not seen to abandon outward shows of deference to black doctors, to direct them to perform specific tasks, to reprimand them for their behaviour, or to openly criticise their professional competence.

Interactional performance and power

Another possible reason for the differences between these two studies is that while the doctors in Hughes' study were not familiar with the cultural cues of the host culture, those in my study were. This is largely the explanation given by Hughes. He argues that their unfamiliarity leads immigrant doctors to be dependent upon nurses for cultural translation, allowing nurses to be far more actively involved in therapy than they would otherwise be. This alteration in the balance of power is exacerbated by the loss of status resulting from nurses observing doctors to 'misconstrue events or omit to make seemingly "obvious" inferences concerning particular cases' (Hughes 1988: 14).

If this explanation is accepted, the differences in power between doctors and nurses in these two studies can be seen in functional terms: those doctors who are competent at their job are given the status usually accorded members of that occupation; those who are perceived as incompetent are not.

What worries me about such an explanation is that it excises the issue of racism altogether, and as we have already seen, racist attitudes were certainly evident in my study at least.

Hughes implicitly deals with racism by introducing Everett Hughes' (1945) concept of status dilemma. Everett Hughes observes that a complex of auxiliary characteristics tend to grow up around a particular status. He identifies whiteness as an auxiliary characteristic of high status occupations such as medicine. A dilemma in status occurs if this expected characteristic is missing. Thus David Hughes explains the relationships he observed in the following terms: 'relations between young, inexperienced Asian [doctors] ... and mature, experienced, Anglo-Saxon nurses almost inevitably involve dilemmas in status, and some departure from expected role relationships' (1988:17).

Though neither of the authors (Hughes 1988 and Hughes 1945) state it, the issue being dealt with here is the effects of a structurally constituted racism. Status is being denied some people because of what others see as their inferior 'racial' characteristics.

It can be seen that David Hughes is positing two separate explanations for the phenomena he observed, one functional and one racialised. He attempts to synthesise these by stating that:

> Everett Hughes's analysis is capable of marriage to contemporary sociological perspectives. Hughes, admittedly, was concerned with contradictions of status primarily in terms of combinations of personal characteristics that violate normative expectations regarding occupational incumbency, but such contradictions are also likely to have direct implications in terms of interactional performance ... [D]ifferential competence in utilizing relevant

bodies of social knowledge is perhaps the most salient interactional manifestation of 'status' characteristics (1988:17-18).

I would argue that the connection between these two factors is only contingent. It may be the case in Hughes' study that 'status differentiation' or, in more critical language, racist discrimination, is mediated through 'differential competence'. However, it would be naive to assume that manifestations of racism are limited to such circumstances. Racism is not suffered exclusively by people who are unattuned to British or Irish culture. The experiences of second and third generation black British people testify to the contrary (Brown 1984).

Nevertheless, the case of members of high status occupations suffering from racism is significant. In Everett Hughes's words:

> membership of the Negro race (sic), as defined in American mores and/or law, may be called a master status-determining trait. It tends to overpower, in most crucial situations, any other characteristic which may run counter to it. But professional standing is also a powerful characteristic ... In the person of the professionally qualified Negro (sic) these two powerful characteristics clash (1945:357).

In other words, there are two contradictory social mechanisms at work here. Racism tends to reduce social status, while professional power enhances it.

The influence of professional ideology

We must now ask why the tendency of racism was latent in my study, but manifest in David Hughes's (1988) study. It will be remembered that Bhaskar (1989b) observes that the actual outcome of a tendency will generally be co-determined by the activity of other mechanisms. In this case, the other mechanism is that of professionalism.

Professional power is based on the ability of professions to maintain occupational closure by such means as credentialism and legal licence (Parkin 1979). These methods of closure in turn depend upon the justificatory ideology of professionalism, central to which are the pattern variables identified by Parsons (1951).

I realise that an attempt to resuscitate Parsonian sociology will be met with some scepticism. However, it is my contention that radical critics of Parsons's theory of professions (for example, Freidson 1970 and Johnson 1972) may have thrown the baby out with the bath water. Turner (1985) has noted that the sociology of professions exemplifies the tendency of the discipline as a whole to lurch from one exaggeration to another. The Parsonian definition of professions emphasised knowledge as the dominant criterion, dismissing the salience of power. In reaction to what they saw as the sanguine naiveté of this position, later commentators asserted that occupational dominance was central, knowledge and ethics being irrelevant. Turner argues that an adequate conception of professions must take both dimensions seriously.

While it may be the case that professional ideology is adopted by professionals for self-serving purposes, namely the maintenance of occupational control, this does not mean that the ideology is non-existent. Notwithstanding the dubiety of its material referent, because ideology has effects it cannot be dismissed as an illusion (Hirst 1979).

It was in his study of the medical profession that Parsons first developed the notion of pattern variables (Holton and Turner 1986). These are of direct relevance to the issue of racism. They are linked together by their emphasis on the importance of rationality. Acceptance of universalistic-achievement values entails doctors being regarded as having attained their occupational status through their ability, independent of ascriptive qualities such as 'race'. Affective neutrality is also pertinent. It assumes that judgements should be made on the basis of scientific rationality rather than affectivity. Similarly, functional specificity only allows doctors to be judged on their skills as doctors, rather than on factors extraneous to the job.

As we saw in Chapter Four, this rationalistic conception of professionalism is largely accepted within the culture of nursing. As a consequence, the variables outlined above are criteria by which actions are judged within the social setting I have described. Naked racism, being irrational, ascriptive, particularistic, diffuse and affective, is therefore not justifiable as an open form of social interaction between nurses and doctors. To be acceptable in this social milieu, racism needs to be cloaked in a 'rational' veneer. This is what is happening when differential competence is married to 'race'. Criticism on the grounds of competence can be portrayed as rational, affectively neutral, universalistic, achievement oriented, and specific to the skills of medicine. Yet, the racism is there. From such a perspective, criticisms of the competence of immigrant doctors can be seen as the vehicle through which racism is expressed. However, the connection between knowledge of social cues and 'race' is not a necessary one. It follows that if a black doctor is culturally literate, an important avenue for the expression of racism is closed off. This does not mean that racism ceases to exist, just that the mechanisms for its articulation are limited - it is submerged in the public arena but continues to find expression backstage. Thus, in a discussion bewailing the infiltration of non-Christian religions, the nurse who deferred publicly to the Palestinian doctor's religious observances but complained about them privately in racist terms (Transcript 7\8), explained her behaviour in the following terms:

Transcript 7\10
Intensive Care Unit

SN(F)1 Why didn't you say something to him about it?

SN(F)2 Well, it wouldn't be proper. It would be a bit unprofessional ...

SN(F)1 It's not exactly professional to get down on your knees in the middle of the clinical ...

SN(F)2   Yea, but you couldn't just say 'Listen you, you're not in Arab land now'.
         I suppose I could have told him that clinical areas have to be open to
         staff at all times.

Connecting structure and agency

To return to critical realism, we can see the complex interpolations that exist
between social structures and social action. While structural racism exists, it is
modified by the professional ideology to which the actors adhere. This counter-
balancing effect is in the nature of open social systems. There is no reason to
suppose that the matrix of structures within which agency occurs will not contain
contradictory elements. Actors are therefore often faced with incongruent structural
variables. This does not imply that actors have total discretion in choosing which
structural tendencies to take notice of and which to ignore; it is possible to
hierarchically rank structures in terms of their explanatory significance for any
specific social event (Bhaskar 1989a).
    Nevertheless, the openness of the social world attenuates the determinant power of
social structures over agency. If structure does not determine action, what then is the
relationship between them?

Rational calculation?

One possible answer to this question is to conceptualise actors as having knowledge
about the constraining and enabling characteristics of the social structures within
which they live, and making conscious choices about what they do, based upon that
knowledge. Thus agents would be seen as being faced with the task of collapsing
structural variables into categories that can inform interactional practices. Goffman
(1983:11) has argued that this is done by means of 'a set of transformational rules,
or a membrane selecting how various externally relevant social distinctions will be
managed within the interaction'. Thus, it could be argued, in a social situation
where nurses deemed open expressions of racism to be inappropriate, they filtered
them out, selecting instead professional modes of interaction.
    This process of filtering out racism in favour of professionalism was encouraged by
the potential victims of that racism. Their success in utilising professionalism to
negate the effects of prejudice varied according to the tactics used. The authoritarian
consultant relied solely on the status ascribed to him by dint of his occupational
position, and did not adopt more subtle justificatory strategies. While his authority
was not formally challenged, it was accepted with bad grace. Onstage, this was
evidenced by the sullen manner by which some nurses interacted with him;
backstage, by the frequency of racist remarks.
    Some indication that this doctor's behaviour was a response to racism was given by
a nurse who had worked in the unit since its foundation:

SR(F)   It's not all his fault. When he came here first he had a hard time of it. People were a bit cheeky. It's not a wonder he closed up.

A more successful strategy was adopted by the knowledgeable doctor. By portraying himself as a paragon of scientific rationality, he was more closely attuned to the presumptions of professionalism, by which the nurses set such store. As a result his authority was not only formally, but also conatively accepted.

While the evidence suggests that some actors, at least, responded to racism in a conscious fashion, this conception of human behaviour is highly rationalistic and calculative. We need to ask whether rationalist explanations are capable of providing a full explanation of racism and its maintenance or transformation by individuals. Certainly, such an interpretation is not without its proponents. One of the strongest versions of this position can be found in rational choice theory (RCT),[4] which has been used to explain racism by a number of commentators, including Banton (1983) and Hechter (1986). For instance, Banton argues that the creation and maintenance of racial boundaries:

> can be illuminated if they are analysed in terms of Rational Choice Theory according to which group members exchange goods and services, seeking their own advantage. If they compete with one another on an individual basis this will tend to dissolve group boundaries. If they compete as groups, their shared interests will lead them to reinforce those boundaries; the whole life and culture of the privileged group will be oriented to defending their exclusive boundary, while the life of the subordinated group will be directed towards the cultivation of their inclusive bonds so as to mobilize strength for the attack upon the practices which exclude them from privilege (1983:136).

Rational choice theory has been criticised on a number of grounds. From within the micro-sociological perspective in which RCT is grounded, Scheff (1992) argues that its exclusive reliance on rationalism means that it fails to recognise the profound importance of emotions in the motivation of human action.

Rex (1986), in a discussion of 'race' and ethnicity, argues that the RCT case is flawed because it fails to fully take account of the fact that individual actions are constrained by the actions or potential actions of others.

At a wider sociological level, Pierre Bourdieu has provided a trenchant critique of RCT. Indeed, his own *theory of practice* can be seen as providing a powerful alternative to rational choice theory's portrayal of the linkage between system and individual.[5] Bourdieu dismisses rational choice theory on the grounds that:

> if one fails to recognize any form of action other than rational action or mechanical reaction, it is impossible to understand the logic of all the actions

that are reasonable without being the product or a reasoned design, still less of rational calculation (1990:50).

One might make this point even more strongly by observing that the belief that rational agency is all that there is certainly cannot explain *unreasonable* actions.

Not every action that human beings perform is the result of prior, conscious, calculation. Much of it is a matter of routine, or 'practical logic', to use Bourdieu's term.[6] We act in certain ways because we regard such actions as 'natural' responses to the stimuli we are faced with - yet they are not 'natural', they are the result of social conditioning as to what is appropriate. For the most part, we do not consider the social construction of our reality, still less the structural mechanisms which predicate that construction - we are, to use Bourdieu's term, in a position of *doxa*.

According to Bourdieu, social actors' performances are predicated upon a shared body of dispositions, which he terms *habitus*. These dispositions are the product of the 'dead weight' of history:

> The *habitus* - embodied history, internalized as a second nature and so forgotten as history - is the active presence of the whole past of which it is the product (Bourdieu 1990:56).

This is not to say that the *habitus* (or, rather, the social structures that produce the habitus) determines human actions. Bourdieu is very careful to talk in terms of dispositions rather than compulsions.[7] Indeed, his aim in developing the concept of habitus is to transcend the antinomy of determinism and freedom. Nor, indeed, does he conceive of practical logic as the only form of logic. Rational choice can be the basis of agency:

> the lines of action suggested by habitus may very well be accompanied by a strategic calculation of costs and benefits ... But, and this is a crucial proviso, it is habitus itself that commands this option. We can always say that individuals make choices, as long as we do not forget that they do not choose the principles of these choices (Bourdieu in Wacquant 1989:45).[8]

In relation to the substantive issue at hand, it might be noted that while the Asian and black doctors in the unit chose to deal with the problem of racism in a variety of ways, their choice of response was limited by the nature of the factor that they were responding to. Racism, and the constrictions upon their lives that it entailed, could not be wished away. The conditions for possible responses were also limited by the occupational milieu in which they worked, in that there are strict limitations to the kind of actions deemed appropriate for physicians. Many of these limitations are organised around the ideology of professionalism. So it can be seen that, while the doctors' responses to the problem of racism were rational, and indeed entailed an effort to optimise their social position (in accordance with rational choice theory), the material circumstances, and the historically generated *habitus* that they worked in, defined the principles of those choices.

135

The case of nurses is more problematical, in that it would seem that they are located in two relatively separate *habiti* - lay and professional. Weber (1968) noted the crucial significance of the separation of place of work and domicile, a division that he regarded as essential to the nature of the modern West. He argued that this separation means that the impersonal ethos of modern bureaucracies can be effectively applied, uncompromised by the affectivities of the private world. According to such logic, racism, being an affective ideology, would have less currency in bureaucratic settings, given their impersonal ethos. Thus, the expression of racism would be more acceptable in the lay *habitus* than in the professional, where it could only occur in disguise.

While the extra-occupational experience of nurses included exposure to racism, their self-image as nurses rested on affective neutrality. This difference was manifested in the contrast between frontstage and backstage behaviours. Frontstage, nurses' discourse was animated by the impersonal professional ethos of the bureaucracy. Backstage, there was a leakage from the lay *habitus*, and as a consequence their discourse contained perspectives whose origins lay outside the occupational domain.

This does not mean that we should conflate nurses' lay culture with their backstage occupational culture. While backstage culture contained lay perspectives, it was also influenced by frontstage occupational *mores*. This was evidenced by the tendency, that I have already noted, for nurses to eschew more blatant species of racist name-calling. Thus, it could be argued that even backstage, professional ideology ensured a degree of 'ideological deracialisation' (to use Reeves's (1983) term), whereby actors' discourse tends to mask the reality of racism, without actually eradicating it.

Nevertheless, some nurses observed backstage in the ICU maintained an almost doxic belief in the acceptability of racist differentiation:

Transcript 7\12
Intensive Care Unit

SN(F) Blacks are a bit that way, though aren't they?

SP That's just racist.

SN(F) No it is not. I can't be blamed if they are that way, nor can they, it's just the way they are.[9]

Despite her firmly held beliefs, this nurse was never heard by me to utter frontstage racist remarks, thus indicating that she adhered to the norms of behaviour associated with occupational ideology. However, from the comment above, we must assume that her adherence to occupational norms did not entail her acceptance of those norms in extra-occupational settings. Racial differences remained a natural part of her lay world and she had no doubt about their reality.

Conversely, the response of Suburban Hospital interviewees indicates that the non-expression of racism in formal occupational settings is part of nurses' doxic experience. When asked about the effect of 'race' upon inter-occupational relations, the nurses denied any such effect:

Transcript 7\13
Medical Ward

SP   Do you think nurses think about black and Asian doctors any differently?

SN(F)   Ehh ... I've never really thought about it. I, ehhh ... no, I don't think so ... maybe you come across a few people who are a bit bigoted, but not that it would make much difference.

Transcript 7\14
Medical Ward

SP   Are nurses ever racist about black or Asian doctors?

SN(F)   Doctors are treated as doctors, not by the colour of their skin.

These responses can be considered in the light of Bourdieu's attacks on the epistemological efficacy of interviews. Bourdieu (1977) argues that when actors do reflect upon their situation, they tend to recount to the researcher what they think ought to be occurring, rather than what is actually occurring. In line with this, I suspect we are seeing in the nurses' avowals an example of the tendency to describe what they think ought to be, rather than what actually is happening. However, I wish to argue that this methodological 'problem' may be used as a virtue rather than a vice. A researcher without knowledge that racism occurs in hospital settings might take these proclamations at face value. However, knowing that it does occur, we can interpret them in a more useful light. What they demonstrate is that open admission of the use of racism without functional pretext within the occupational setting is not acceptable, in that the taint of racism will devalue nurses' professional standing. This further reinforces the impression that professional ideology, and the institutions that embody it, provide a powerful and distinctive *habitus*.

The empirical material presented here, in itself, cannot tell us whether the nurses interviewed were consciously dissimulating or whether their statements represented 'practical logic' generated by the occupational *habitus*. In support of the latter interpretation, I certainly gained the impression that my interviewees were not deliberately attempting to pull the wool over my eyes, and that their protestations were made in good faith.

Thus, it would seem that lay and professional *habiti* can contain contradictory assumptions without actors having to directly and consciously having to address those contradictions. This absence of rational uniformity should not be seen as surprising, for as Gramsci observes, 'common sense is an ambiguous, contradictory and multiform concept' (1971:423).

The complexity of racism

It can be seen that the effects of structural racism upon the attitudes of white nurses, and on their relations with black and Asian doctors were extremely convoluted. I have argued that the racist dispositions of some nurses, as articulated in backstage encounters, did not determine their actions in frontstage dealings with doctors. One of the reasons for this disjuncture between disposition and practice was that nurses were experiencing the generative effects of two countervailing social mechanisms, namely racism and professionalism.

While racist attitudes were a normal part of the lay worlds of some nurses, it was not acceptable for them to act in an openly racist fashion within their formal occupational milieu, unless they could cloak those actions in a 'rational' veneer. This was because racism offended against the rationalist ethos of professionalism, an ideology highly valued by nurses.

The example of racism shows us just how complex the relationship between social structures and individual agency actually is.

Notes

1. 'Racialised groups' is the term used by Miles (1982) to describe those groups to which the ideological category of 'race' has been attributed. He uses the term to emphasise that the concept of 'race' emerges from ideology rather than biology.
2. The existence of Irish racism is testament to the complexities of structural relationships, confounding mono-causal explanations which exclusively locate racism in the economics of imperialism and its aftermath. This theoretically awkward phenomenon has, up until recently, received little attention. However, McVeigh (1992) has proposed a five point aetiology of Irish racism: the diffusion of racism from Britain, the influence of the Diaspora, the involvement of Irish people in Western imperialism, the grafting of racism onto sectarianism, and the existence of endogenous anti-Traveller racism.
3. In fairness to the nurses, racist language was rarely uttered. Nevertheless, the fact that a few nurses felt able to use it with impunity indicates that racism was at least tolerated in backstage culture.
4. The distinctive features of rational choice theory have been described by Coleman and Fararo. they categorise it as 'a theory of transitions between the level of social system behavior and the level of behavior of individual actors' (1992:ix). According to Coleman and Fararo, the unique contribution of RCT lies in its emphasis on the calculative element in human behaviour:

> Rational choice theory contains one element that differentiates it from nearly all other theoretical approaches in sociology. This element can be

summed up in a single word: *optimization*. The theory specifies that in acting rationally, an actor is engaging in some kind of optimization ... [I]t is this that gives rational choice theory its power: It compares actions according to their expected outcomes for the actor and postulates that the actor will choose the action with the best outcome (1992:xi).

5. Inclusion of Bourdieu's theory of practice is necessary because of a significant explanatory gap in Bhaskar's critical realism. While Bhaskar demonstrates convincingly (to my mind) that social structures exist, and that they provide the means, media, rules and resources upon which human agency is founded, he is less detailed in his discussion of *how* they do so. He simply identifies 'socialisation' as the point of articulation from structure to agency, and makes little further comment. Bourdieu's theory of practice has the merit of providing a fuller theorisation of this problematic.

6. The idea of practical logic has strong echoes of Schutz's concept of 'natural attitude', whereby actors, for the most part, suspend doubt about the social world and regard its appearance as solid reality. However, Schutz overly privileges subjectivity. For him, the social world is 'essentially only something dependent upon and still within the operating intentionality of ego-consciousness' (1967:44). Thus, causality flows *from* the natural attitude *to* the social world. Giddens (1976) has criticised Schutz's phenomenology on the grounds that it cannot take account of either unacknowledged effects of actions, or of determining conditions that are not mediated by the consciousness of the actor.

7. This is consistent with Bhaskar's insistence that laws can only be analysed as tendencies, and not as constant conjunctions.

8. Once again, Bourdieu's thesis is consistent with the tenets of critical realism. It will be remembered that Bhaskar observes that while 'We do not create society - the error of voluntarism' (1989a:3), it is also the case that 'society does not exist independently of human agency - the error of reification' (1989a:4).

9. This strategy of presenting racist statements as objective observations is similar to that used by the nurse in transcript 7\6. These attempts to co-opt rationality to justify the irrational is evidence that even backstage, rationalist *mores* have a powerful influence.

8 Capitalism

Introduction

The purpose of this chapter is to examine how the nature of capitalism affects inter-occupational relations within public health care institutions. The discussion will be framed along the lines of a broadly Marxist analysis, in that it will concentrate on the influence of the economic base upon the position of nursing and medicine. Belief that such an influence exists is founded upon the assumption that the trajectory along which the welfare state develops corresponds at least partially to the changes in the patterns of capitalist economic accumulation.

Following the long post-war boom, upon which the growth of the welfare state was based, capitalist accumulation has been in a state of crisis since the early 1970s (Currie 1983). It rapidly became accepted that the orthodox Keynesian response of using increased public expenditure to pull capitalist economies back into health would not work again (Gough 1983). Indeed one of the major problems facing western economies was the drag upon the rate of profit that resulted from the proportion of gross domestic product that was being soaked up by the state (O'Connor 1976).

The response to the crisis of capitalism has been along two, closely interrelated lines. The first was to attempt to solve the fiscal crisis of the state by reducing the proportion of GNP that found its way into the coffers of the welfare state. The battle to reduce spending on the welfare state has been an explicit, and overriding concern of British Conservative Governments since 1979.

A more diffuse response to the crisis of capital accumulation came in the form of the reorganisation (or disorganisation - cf. Lash and Urry 1987) of systems of production and consumption. The traditional form of production, known as Fordism, entailed the mass production of standardised products, using flowline assembly, and dedicated machinery (Murray 1989a).[1] The inflexibility inherent in this form of production translated itself into a lack of choice for consumers. In an effort to improve rate of profit, capitalist production has been undergoing a phase of reconstruction, known as post-Fordism, which, in relation to industry consists of applying computer technology not only to each stage of the production process, from design to retailing, but also to the integration of all stages of the process into a single co-ordinated system. As a result, the economies of scale of mass production can now be achieved on much smaller runs ... Instead of Fordism's specialised machinery producing standardised products, we now have flexible, all-purpose machinery producing a variety of products ... Distribution has been revolutionised, as has the link between sales, production and innovation (Murray 1989b:56-7).

Nor is post-Fordism restricted to industrial production. The same sort of functional flexibility has been introduced into service industries and nursing is no exception. Nursing reforms can be interpreted as an example of this new mode of production. Walby *et al.* (1994) identify three developments of nursing which enhance the flexibility of nursing work. First, Project 2000 training, which entails higher standards of academic education and the inculcation of more general principles, will enable nurses trained in this programme to have more discretion in their responses to patients' requirements than the more regimented form of training that it has replaced allowed for. Second, the development of primary nursing entails the rejection of task-orientation in favour of more individualised forms of care. Third, the UKCC's (1922a) assertion that the basis of nurses' accountability should be the Council's principles of practice rather than the accumulation of certificates, entails a move away from an inflexible   rule-focused approach to one where individual judgement provides the basis for decision making.

However, we need to be beware of exaggerating the pervasiveness of post-Fordism. Fordist forms of production continue to co-exist with it (Lipietz 1987; Crompton 1993). Specifically, there is no reason to suppose that changes in capitalist production will automatically be read off in changes to the organisation of welfare services such as the NHS (Rustin 1989). As Walby *et al.* (1994) observe, recent developments in the health service are not a matter of simple transition from the logic of Fordism to that of post-Fordism, but rather an uneasy co-existence of both. On the one hand, there is pressure upon hospitals to maximise the number of patients treated, on the other hand, there is the rhetoric of individualised care. Walby *et al.* concluded from their study that:

There was a contradiction between the desire for higher throughput typical of Taylorist management and a Fordist regime, and the patient-centred, ward-based, cohesive interprofessional team more appropriate to new wave management and post-Fordism. If the patient, as consumer, is the centre with individuated packages of care, then Taylorist management is inappropriate. The tension between these coexisting logics of organisation was evident in many issues in the hospital (1994:158).

The manner in which capitalism impacts upon nurse-doctor relations is different to that of patriarchy, racism or sectarianism. In the latter cases, segments of the different groups were clearly aligned along gender, 'race' and sect fractures. In the case of class, the situation is more ambiguous.

Looking at nurses' relationship with the means of production, it is fairly clear that they are neither in a position of ownership nor control, and can therefore be defined, in Marxist terms, as part of the proletariat. Doctors are less easy to place. A reductive Marxist definition might well place them in the proletariat along with nurses - if we exclude private practice, as salaried employees of the state, doctors do not enjoy ownership of the means of production with which they labour. However, the issue of control is far less clear, leading to wide differences in the interpretations of commentators.

Some Marxists such as Navarro (1978) argue that health care structures cannot be internally explained through examination of the forces within medicine. Rather, the shape that health care takes results from the class relations that pertain. From such a perspective, the medical profession is seen as little more than a stooge of capitalism, serving its interests through ideological justification and social control.

Contrary to this position, neo-Weberians like Freidson (1970) argue that, while professions such as medicine may have emerged by the 'grace of powerful protectors' (1972:xii), they have succeeded in gaining considerable autonomy from such groups, at least in terms of the technical control of their work. Indeed, it is this autonomy that defines them as 'professions'.

A third position is taken by Terence Johnson (1993) who argues that professions emerged neither as servants of, nor independent from, the state, but as an integral part of the apparatus that constitutes the modern state. Following Foucault (1979), Johnson argues that power is closely interlocked with knowledge. In the modern era, the power\knowledge duality entails the classification and surveillance of populations, and the normalisation and disciplining of individuals. The establishment of the jurisdiction of professions such as medicine, law and psychiatry was consequent upon the problems of government that emerged in the nineteenth century. It was these groups that supplied the expert knowledge essential for power. Johnson observes that the implications of his argument are that:

> we must develop ways of talking about state and profession that conceive of the relationship not as a struggle for autonomy or control but as the interplay of integrally related structures, evolving as the combined product of occupational strategies, governmental policies, and shifts in public opinion (1993:12).

Johnson's Foucauldian model of the state has little to say about the state's relation to the economic base. However, it is possible to combine the sort of complex structural interaction model that Johnson is advocating with an acceptance of the importance of class structure upon the nature of the welfare state. Such a line is taken by Miliband (1973) in his portrayal of the state as consisting of groups of mutually supportive elites, all of whom share a basic interest in the preservation of capitalism.

Whether we interpret the medicine as a buffer which acts to 'increase the social security and power of the upper ten thousand' (Marx 1969:573), as an autonomous profession, or as part of the power\knowledge matrix, one thing is clear: doctors' position within capitalism has been considerably more powerful than that enjoyed by nursing. However, there are signs that things may be changing.

The decline of medicine?

While elite professions such as medicine may be more closely tied to the state than some Marxist and neo-Weberian commentators allow, this does not mean that the relationship between different elite groups should be seen as static. There is a degree of consensus that recent developments within the constellation of social elites have been to the disadvantage of the medical profession.

Bureaucratisation

The relative decline of medicine is often explained in terms of the shift in its locus of practice. Most doctors now work within a bureaucratic setting. Consequently, the occupation has had to adjust of the exigencies of bureaucracy, and to come to an accommodation with administrators. For example, McKinlay and Arches (1985) argue that bureaucratisation of health care, resulting from the demands of advanced capitalism, has lead to the steady proletarianisation of physicians.[2] While they conceive of professions as being separated from the rest of the capitalist state, it is possible to combine their analysis with that of Johnson by observing that recent developments in the organisation of advanced capitalism have tended to lead to the empowerment of administrative elites to the cost of elite groups possessing technical expertise. The degree to which this shift in power has actually occurred is a matter for empirical adjudication. As we shall see, there is evidence that the retreat of doctors in the face of bureaucratic encroachment has been more apparent than real.

De-skilling

The proletarianisation of professions such as medicine has also been projected in terms of technologically driven de-skilling (Haug 1973; Oppenheimer 1973). This thesis has recently been revived in discussions about new technologies. Thus, for example, Gershuny and Miles (1983) have identified a number of techniques, such as computer-aided diagnostics and remote monitoring using telecommunications, which could radically change the nature of health care services.

However, once again there is evidence that the effect of technological innovations upon the status of doctors has not been as dramatic as might have been expected. Child (1986) has argued that doctors have successfully deflected the threat to their occupational position posed by new information technologies. Their professional status, the 'indeterminacy' of their knowledge base (cf. Jamous and Peloille 1970), the nature of their relationship with patients, and the fact that they have considerable control over the course and content of technological changes, have all contributed to the ability of doctors to defend their position in relation to new technology.

An example of the ability of doctors to maintain their occupational standing, despite technologically driven changes in work practices can be seen in Harvey's (1987) examination of anaesthetists' relationships with intensive care nurses. Despite the fact that these nurses operate advanced technology as an intrinsic part of their job, and have therefore experienced considerable 'up-skilling', they have not broken out of nurse-doctor relations that pertain in other specialities.

Gender and de-skilling

Harvey explains the continued subordinate position of intensive care nurses in terms of the sex-typing of their occupation. This serves as a reminder that there are dangers in separating the various structural mechanisms that pertain in specific social situations. The effects of these structures are often intimately linked.

The conceptualisation and measurement of skill is, at least in part, a social process (Crompton 1987). Specifically, the gender of workers will have a critical influence upon the degree of skill that their occupational tasks are accredited with (Phillips and Taylor 1980).

It may be that the alteration in the gender balance of medicine has had some effect upon social perceptions of doctors' skills. As Rees notes, 'Feminisation of a particular occupation or profession is seen to have the effect of deskilling it' (1992:16). Certainly, women entering medicine have been channelled away from those specialities, such as surgery, which enjoy the reputation of entailing high levels of technological skill and dexterity (Oliver and Walford 1991). Whether or not the increasing numbers of women in medicine has had an effect on the social construction of medical skill *in toto* is difficult to ascertain. However, once again, it is wise to be cautious about the degree of change that has occurred. Occupations are normally sex-typed during the process of their formation. Once that sex-typing has taken place, it is highly resistant to change (Crompton 1987; Milkman 1983; Murgatroyd 1982).

Post-Fordist flexibility

Technological innovation, and the flexibility of production that it allows is one aspect of post-Fordism. Another aspect of post-Fordist flexibility is the development of new consumption norms. In relation to health care, this development has taken a number of paths, including the commodification of personal preventative health care such as exercise and diet (Jessop 1991), the development of mass-consumption markets for health care products that bypass formal health services (Blackburn *et al.* 1985), the increasing popularity of 'alternative' forms of health care (Sharma 1990), and the expansion of private health care insurance provision (Dunleavy and

Husbands 1985). Nursing's attempts to expand out of its traditional role can also be viewed in terms of the increasing flexibility of health care consumption. While it is difficult to quantify precise effects of post-Fordism on the position of doctors, all these developments, with the possible exception of the privatisation of medical care, tend to undermine the occupational position of doctors, who formally enjoyed almost monopoly control over the consumption of health care services.

Fiscal crisis and administrative controls

Another trend that has been identified as having a deleterious effect upon the position of medicine is the expansion of political controversy into areas of decision-making that were once seen as the exclusive and neutral arena of medical experts (Starr and Immergut 1987). The fiscal crisis of the state from the 1970s on, focused governmental attention on the costs of public expert services. Health care services came under particular scrutiny because issues of cost were exacerbated by demographic trends, notably the increasing proportion of elderly people in the population. One of the tactics used to rein in health care expenditure levels was to restrict the autonomy of doctors by subjecting them to auditing and monitoring systems.

While this trend can be traced at least as far back as the Labour government decision in 1976 to abandon 'demand-led' expenditure on the health services in favour of cash limits (see Allsop 1984), it reached fruition in the Thatcher era, during which there were a number of attempts to radically alter the organisation and jurisdiction of expert services such as medicine. Thus the 1980s saw an almost continual stream of measures that were aimed at reforming the organisation of the NHS. The most important of these were the introduction of a general managerial system following the Griffiths Report (1983) and the changes that occurred as a result of the reforms that emerged from the *Working for Patients* (1989) White Paper.

The managerial reforms that occurred following Griffiths entailed a reduction in the power of clinical managers. The previous system of managing through the medically dominated consensus of professions was abandoned. In its stead was placed a general managerial system which was strategically driven by central governmental directives, and which, it was hoped, would be powerful enough to override medical objections to financial rationalisation. In short, the introduction of general management could be seen as a challenge to medical dominance within the NHS (Cox 1992).

The results were not as dramatic as the government might have hoped for. In a review of post-Griffiths management changes, Harrison concludes that although 'the frontier of control between government and doctors has shifted a little, in favour of the former, there is as yet little evidence that managers have secured greater control over doctors' (1988:122).

While the formal changes appeared to be radical, medical control over clinical activity remained largely undisturbed (Harrison *et al.* 1990). The ineffectiveness of these reforms was recognised by government, which drafted the proposals contained in *Working for Patients* with the aim of completing unfinished business. It was argued in the White Paper that 'the government believes that it is unacceptable for local management to have little authority or influence over ... [consultants] who are in practice responsible for committing most of the hospital services' resources' (cited Butler 1992:40).

The new strategy hoped to constrain the clinical autonomy of consultants, and to tie them more closely to the managerial system through the negotiation of new contracts. A financial stick to enforce the new arrangements was provided by the freedom of the new hospital trusts to formulate their own terms and conditions for hospital staff (Butler 1992).

Organisational reforms and nursing

It is ironic that while commentators tend to identify the motivations of the health service reforms with the attempt by government to reduce the clinical autonomy of doctors, it is probable that the reforms have had a greater effect upon the position of nursing.

The Griffiths reforms had an especially traumatic effect. The Royal College of Nursing fought a bitter, expensive, and in the end fruitless campaign in the press to prevent loss of nursing control over nurses. Despite its efforts, the reforms cut swathes through nursing management. While the nature of work at Ward Sister\Charge Nurse level was initially little affected, the stress and disillusionment experienced in response to Griffiths was felt throughout the occupation (Owens and Glennerster 1990).

It might be thought that as well as bringing in outside control over nurses, the general management system would have given nurses the opportunity to gain control over areas of health service management beyond the nursing remit. However, evidence of Owens and Glennerster's (1990) study of one regional health authority indicates that nurses did not enjoy this compensation. Physicians refused to accept the authority of those nurses who were appointed to the new service managerial posts, continuing to view their relations in traditional terms. Physicians' resentment of and resistance to management intervention meant that managers who were nurses felt that they lacked any real authority or control.

However, there is evidence that in the decade since the Griffiths Report, senior nurses have become increasingly comfortable with the general managerial system. The number of general managers with a nursing background has increased from 35 in 1986 to 120 in 1993 (Brindle 1993). An example of the change of heart experienced by nurses can be found in Ray Rowden, who was centrally involved in the RCN's advertising campaign to oppose implementation of general management, and who now describes it as 'the best thing that ever happened' (cited in Brindle 1993:15). One of its advantages, according to Rowden, is that it has smashed through the tribal barriers surrounding nurses and doctors.

While the effects of organisational reforms were initially felt at nursing managerial level, they have increasingly impinged on the role of the Ward Sister, which has expanded in many cases to take on budgetary as well as care responsibilities. With the decimation of middle management in the form of nursing officers, senior clinical nurses have become an integral part of the new managerial system (Jones 1990).

The practical effects of organisational reforms

The literature indicates that alterations in the form and requirements of the economic base, as mediated through governmental directives, have impinged upon the relative positions of medicine and nursing in a number of ways. The extent of the changes, however, has been the subject of debate. Empirical testing of the degree to which changes in the organisation of health care provision has changed the occupational position of nursing and its relation to medicine can be gained from examination of the situation in Suburban Hospital. Three approaches to the question will be taken here:

1.   The effects of managerial reforms upon the organisation of nursing.

2.   The effects of managerial reforms upon the organisation of medicine.

3.   The effects of post-Fordist flexibility upon inter-occupational relations.

Managerial reforms and nursing

Evidence from Suburban Hospital indicated that the role of the Ward Sister has changed significantly in recent years. The primary locus of the Sister's role had moved away from organising the day-to-day care of patients, towards a wider planning and administrative role.

A clear indication that the Ward Sister's function had altered was given to me when I went to interview the Sister in charge of the medical unit. The interview took place on an empty ward, soon to become a brand new medical facility. The reason for having the interview there, rather than on the ward that was currently being used, was that it was the Sister's responsibility to commission the equipment for the new unit. The strategic task of commissioning was taking up a considerable proportion of the Sister's time. Along with other administrative duties, it meant that the time she had left to spend on first-line management, never mind direct patient care, was severely constrained

Transcript 8\1
Medical Unit

SR(F)   I try very hard to keep as close a contact as I can with the ward work, but it is becoming more and more difficult. Between committees, audit exercises and the rest, the time is just eaten up. I can literally go for days without setting foot on the ward. I can't say I like it much, but I'm afraid it's the sign of the times, ward managers, not sisters.

One of the results of the administrative elevation of ward sisters has been a corresponding elevation of the administrative role of staff nurses. A rough formula might be that sisters have taken over many of the tasks previously performed by nursing officers; senior staff nurses have stepped into the roles shed by sisters; and junior staff nurses and, to some extent, enrolled nurses are doing jobs once done by more senior staff nurses.

Transcript 8\2
Medical Unit

SP   So, who is doing the day-to-day stuff that used to be your job?

SR(F)   [F grade staff nurse] and the other senior staff nurses are in charge of most of the day-to-day running now. Mostly, they have an administrative, not a care role now. With the few staff, they have to do what they can with the patients, but it's their job to make sure that the ward keeps running from one day to the next.

The increased responsibility of junior nurses is also a result of the emergence of primary nursing, whereby, rather than the nurse in charge of the ward directing the care of all the patients on that ward, nurses with sufficient experience are each given primary responsibility for a small number of patients.

These changes have had significant ramifications as far as relations between doctors and junior nurses are concerned. Traditionally, doctors of all ranks dealt almost exclusively with ward sisters or senior staff nurses. Even if their requests and orders impinged upon the work of more junior nursing staff, they were still filtered through the nursing ranks from the nurse in charge downwards. This sort of aloof authority enhanced the power of doctors over less senior nursing staff.

It is no longer simply sisters and senior staff nurses that have the opportunity to discuss issues with their medical colleagues. Doctors are now obliged to communicate with primary nurses.

Transcript 8\3
Surgical Unit

SR(F)   I feel that since primary nursing has started here, we have obviously had a few problems in trying to get the medical staff to understand what we are trying to do, but over the few years that we have been ongoing, I think it has worked and hopefully ... they would know who to go to as a primary nurse, who to get information from. My own personal role - I wouldn't always go on a ward round if I was here. The ward sister\ward manager's role has developed in such a way that time isn't always on our side, therefore I feel that the nurses who are primary nurses and who have developed that role are very competent. I wouldn't let them take on the role if I didn't feel that. So the consultants have to deal with the first line of nurses and not the ward sister all the time.

SP So within nursing itself there has been a delegation of clinical responsibility?

SR(F) I feel that there has been and I do think there will be more because with the way constraints are going and the extra input that is being put on to the ward manager\ward co-ordinator, it isn't always possible for them to be at the bedside. Now, having said that, I personally believe that I, as a ward manager and as a clinical practitioner must maintain my clinical expertise, and I can still do that as a teacher and a facilitator, but it isn't possible for me to have the same input in the clinical area as I had before. Time doesn't permit. Physically, it is just not possible.

Not only have these developments given junior nurses a voice in decision-making, they have also increased the influence of ward sisters in the higher administrative echelons.

Transcript 8\4
Surgical Unit

SP Do you think you now have more influence at a strategic level within the hospital than you did as a traditional ward sister?

SR(F) I think it is going that way. I think obviously it has a long way to go but I do feel that, yes, I have been involved, consulted before change has taken place. However, whether that change would have taken place without my opinion being put forward, I don't know, but I know that within the general management structure, management are more open to suggestion and they are more open to listen to you than they were before.

It can be seen that, despite the fears of nurses when reforms of the administration of the NHS were first introduced, there is evidence that they have improved the position of clinical nurses. Previously, senior doctors were the only clinical staff to enjoy an input into administrative structures concerned with strategic planning. Ward sisters are now gaining an *entree* into these rarefied strata of decision-making. Correspondingly, junior nursing staff are no longer expected to silently obey medical orders as relayed to them by their nursing managers.

SN(F)   No, things have changed. Sister isn't around, I don't mean she isn't working, she works very hard, but she's got to do her management duties which means she can't be doing other things. We would do the round now for our primary patients. It means that we have much more to do with the consultants. Before it would just be Sister on the round and she'd inform us of the consultants orders after. Now we do it. I think it is far better because they are actually dealing with the nurses that are providing the care. We know all the details that you get from being with a patient all day.

SP   Do you think that being on the round yourself gives you more decisions-making power?

SN(F)   I think it must do because at least the consultant gets to hear what you think. Whether he takes any heed of it or not is another matter. But before, you didn't even have the chance to tell him your opinions about care or the patients condition, unless you had asked the Sister to say something. I'm not sure about more power, but we certainly have more influence from being on the rounds.

It is not simply in their interactions with doctors that junior nurses status has been enhanced. They also have more autonomy in their dealings with patients and relatives. Previously the tendency was that if any difficulty arose, the automatic response was to refer the issue immediately to the nurse in charge. Now, nurses feel that they have the remit to tackle problems themselves.

Transcript 8\6
Surgical Unit

SP   A number of nurses have told me that they are taking on more responsibilities that used to be shouldered by Sister. Do you think that this has occurred here?

EN(F)   I think it has here, definitely. Nurses are much more responsible now. They feel much more involved with their care. Plus the relatives - before you always referred all the relatives to your nurse in charge, whereas now if you're acting as a primary or associate nurse, you deal with it and if you've any problems, you know that the manager is always there if you need her. There is much more involvement.

SN(F)   The relatives will actually come looking for you. It gives the primary nurse that wee bit more autonomy.

SP   But it would be delegation within nursing rather than an expansion of nursing as a whole?

EN(F)   I don't know. I think it makes the primary nurses more aware of the whole treatment and care, not just task allocation - you do this and you do that and everything will be OK. You really look at the patient more holistically. You look at them, their family, you do take everybody into consideration. You get more job satisfaction too.

SN(F)   And the patients actually like ... You'll hear them 'Oh, here's my nurse now'.

EN(F)   There has been a change in the patients, definitely, you know. They appreciate the closer relationship. They're not so afraid to ask questions. They know that you have now time to sit down with them and Sister will not be running round to see what I'm doing sitting down with them. You can explain everything to them and you feel that they ask more questions now, don't they?

SN(F)   Uh huh, I think a lot has to do with our ward sister. She has been prepared to step down and act as ward co-ordinator and let you get with it. She'll advise you, but she'll not tell you what to do. I think that may have something to do with our relationship with JHOs. If you know five patients well, you would be more inclined to act as advocate for them because they are your five patients. Whereas if you had 25, you mightn't be inclined to bother so much.

The final comment here highlights the intimate connection between changes in nurse-doctor relations and nurse-patient relations. Closer identification with patients has led to a greater preparedness to challenge doctors on their behalf.

Managerial reforms and medicine

On the medical side, there was little evidence that managerial reforms had significantly affected the position of doctors in the administrative hierarchy. It may have been the case that relations between administrators and doctors *had* altered, but this did not impinge significantly on nurse-doctor dynamics.

Transcript 8\7
Medical Unit

SP   With the new management systems that are being put into place, do you notice any difference in the role of doctors?

SN(F)   Not that I can think of. I think maybe [Consultant] has more on his plate, but it doesn't really have much to do with us. I think it is nurses that have borne the brunt of extra paper work and admin. As usual, the doctors have got off lightly.

Transcript 8\8
Medical Unit

SP   Do you think management changes have had any effect on the way that [Consultant] deals with you?

SR(F)   From his side? I don't think so. From my side, I think I am probably involved in things now that he might have dealt with on his own at one time, but that's about the height of it.

It should be stressed that the evidence presented here is filtered through a nursing perspective, and therefore may well provide a very limited picture. It is unwarranted to extrapolate that, because nurses have not noticed a radical alteration in the role of doctors as a result of administrative reforms, alteration has not occurred. However, the fact that its ramifications are not visible to members of an occupation working closely with medicine, would tend to indicate that change remains circumscribed.

The effects of flexibility

It has already been noted that developments such as primary nursing can be interpreted as part of the move towards post-Fordist working practices. The starkest example of the advance of post-Fordist flexibility in the Suburban Hospital was found in the recently inaugurated Nursing Development Unit (NDU). As the name suggests, the care on this unit was centred around nursing, rather than medicine. This did not mean that doctors were excluded, nor that they were relieved of any of their formal responsibilities. However, it did mark a clear break from the traditional organisation of hospital care, where consultants were seen as the central players in organising admission, treatment and discharge. In the NDU, nurses were given the opportunity to be much more involved in the organisation of these facets of care.

The opening of the unit was a recognition that medically-centred care was not the only appropriate model of institutionalised health care. It was also a recognition that the freeing up of the health care market, most notably through general practitioners gaining control of their budgets, meant that the forms of care that hospitals had on offer needed to be sufficiently flexible to meet market demands. According to the Unit Co-Ordinator, it was the exigencies of the market economy that persuaded senior medical staff to go along with the setting up of such a unit.

Transcript 8\9
Nursing Development Unit

SP   The consultants must have been involved in the idea of a nursing development unit, so are they committed?

UC(F)   They saw it as one way of selling their beds. In this day and age, the way fundholding is organised, the idea that they can say to GPs 'We've a nursing development unit' is good for them, and let's face it, that's the way medical staff have to think now.

While senior medics were prepared to allow such a unit to set up, they may not have been aware of the consequences that their decision would have in terms of their authority over nursing and other health care occupations.

Transcript 8\10
Nursing Development Unit

UC(F)   Just after we moved into the NDU, we had a team building exercise for representatives of all disciplines, and that was where we sat down as a group and discussed our roles and how it fitted into the unit, and discussed other roles, and how I saw the role of the consultant was not how he saw his role, where he was the head of the unit and the controlling body, and made major decisions regarding admission and discharge. He certainly makes decisions about admission, although he now gives us an opportunity - you know, he'll present the patient that is going to come in and ask do we think we can offer this person something, because in the early days we had inappropriate referrals and we just went to the consultant and said 'What are you playing at? This is a complete waste of a bed. We can't offer this patient something. They can go to the day hospital. They can go to such-and-such.' Within two days of him saying 'I'm not letting you dictate completely, but I accept what you're saying', the patient's discharged. Well, that went on for a while until he realised that it would be better to have us in on the process from the start.

While nurses were still careful not to overstep the mark their dealings with consultants in terms of professional etiquette, they were well aware that the balance of power had shifted significantly in their favour. In the NDU it was nurses who decided when medical intervention was required, and not doctors who decided when nursing intervention was required.

153

UC(F) The consultants both here see themselves as the head of the team, but in fact all they do is they admit patients to the unit. They are the doorkeepers. They let people in. Once the patient comes to us, then the most prominent roles are the nursing, the physio [physiotherapy] and the OT [occupational therapy], because the consultant visits the ward once a week. Medical staff are called upon as a problem arises. If somebody's blood pressure is such-and-such, the doctor is called in to discuss that, to see if medication or further tests are required. Or if there is difficulty with patients' behaviour, our medical staff here still have to refer the patient to the clinical psychologist, or the psychiatrist. It can't come through us. Therefore, they are sometimes a bit of a go between. We are identifying the problem, we are passing it on to them and they pass it on to somebody else.

The degree to which nurses on the unit have pushed their agenda can be seen from the way they have gained control over discharge.

Transcript 8\12
Nursing Development Unit

UC(F) Never will the doctor say 'The patient can go home on Friday' Now, sometimes they will still try, and say 'Well, maybe he's ready for home next week', and the chances are that they will get balled out by either a nurse, a physio or a social worker - 'Yes, we will get the patient home when such-and-such has been installed in the house and when so-and-so has done such-and-such.' So what our consultants now do is they say 'Should we aim for the end of March or the end of April?' and the team will probably say 'Yes, that's fair enough' but when it comes to the date of discharge, the primary nurse will organise that date, once she has had feedback from social work, physio and OT to say 'Right, the home help's ready to move in. The rails in the bathroom have been installed. They are now able to walk upstairs.' And then they negotiate with the patient and the family. All these things have been put into operation and we say 'We're ready if you're ready' and then they negotiate. Sometimes you find that where families are involved, if there's a daughter working or whatever, they might plan to take time off work, so you might have to hold a patient for a week until they can get that organised.

In terms of this study, the Nursing Development Unit is exceptional. It is the only unit where nursing autonomy has been advanced significantly along formal lines. Whether it is a portent of things to come, or an anomaly, is a matter of conjecture.

In support of the former thesis, it might be argued that it has simply entailed the fixing of relationships that exist in a more fluid form in other units. Thus, the move from informal to formal involvement in decision-making could be seen as another stage in the progressive development of nursing from a subordinate to an autonomous occupation.

A less optimistic interpretation would highlight the type of patient and the nature of the care carried out on the Nursing Development Unit. The majority of patients looked after in the NDU are elderly. The purpose of the unit is to rehabilitate them, in order to ready them for a return to the community. Typically, they come to the NDU from traditional, medically dominated wards, where they had been looked after during the acute phase of their illness.

Both the type of patient, and the type of problem that leads them to need care, are often seen by doctors as 'unglamorous'. Crucially, these patients no longer require heroic intervention, but often need considerable amounts of 'basic' care. We saw in Chapter Five that doctors, because they regarded psychological care of patients as peripheral to their treatment, were prepared to allow nurses a degree of autonomy in dealing with patients' anxieties. The same could be said of much of the care that is carried out in the NDU. The sort of work carried out in the unit has traditionally been seen by doctors as low-technology, labour-intensive and of low status - in short, nursing work. The medical role in the care and rehabilitation of the elderly has tended to be little more than supervisory. Apart from the prescription of medication, there is little that doctors actually do for elderly patients. Thus, the novelty of the NDU lies in nurses being given the opportunity to supervise themselves, rather than in their taking over clinical activities previously the remit of doctors.

Summary

On examining the empirical effects of the changing nature of the economic base upon the organisation of working practices within health care institutions, we can approach the issue from two directions.

Firstly, we can examine the consequences of attempts to tackle the fiscal crisis of the state by tightening control over health care expenditure. There was little evidence that governmental attempts to restrict the clinical autonomy of doctors had a significant direct impact upon their occupational position. However, the quality of nurse-doctor interactions *was* altered by the impact that managerial reforms had upon nurses. The eradication of a middle-management tier in nursing administration meant that the administrative responsibilities of grades beneath middle management tended to be increased. This in turn meant that junior clinical nurses who previously had little direct access to doctors became part of the interactive process.

Secondly, we can consider how the tendency towards more flexible styles of work organisation have affected the standing of medicine and nursing. We can conclude that in many areas, there is little evidence of the advent of post-Fordism. While nursing discretion and involvement in decision-making may have increased, traditional divisions of labour remain largely intact. However, the case of the

Nursing Development Unit is a significant exception to this rule. The NDU can be seen as an example of medical retrenchment in the face of pressures to cut back its expensive monopoly. It may be true that the ground medicine has given is the ground that it least values. Nevertheless, its tactical retreat in this instance is real enough. At the very least, the opening of Nursing Development Units signals an acceptance by medicine that the area which it can claim exclusively as its own will be smaller than that to which it previously had pretentions. This acceptance allows nursing to expand its role along autonomous lines.

The downside of post-Fordism

One should not be too sanguine about the 'restructuring' of the welfare state. While some of those nurses still in work may be in a stronger position *vis-à-vis* doctors, most nurses have paid a heavy price for this advantage in terms of either work-overload or unemployment.

In the Health and Social Services Board within which Metropolitan Hospital was located, hospital admissions rose by 8% between 1981 and 1988\9, while nursing staffing levels fell by 6% between 1982 and 1989 (Eastern Health and Social Services Board 1992). One of the consequences of increased work loads is that more time-consuming, New Nursing aspects of care tend to be overlooked in favour of getting through the basic tasks required of nurses, as the following transcript clearly indicates:

Transcript 8\13
Medical Ward

SP   Primary nursing is ...

SN(F)   It's a title. We have a board out there. We are responsible for so many patients, but, again, the time factor of actually going round different patients, your patients - your five or seven patients every day - it's very difficult (...)

SP   Is that just because you're in charge?

SN(F)   No, I would say that's a general problem for everyone. The turnover is so much higher than it was years ago. You are not really managing. I feel we are always on coping level. This ward used to run with maybe seven and eight staff,[3] and at its worst day it was six and seven. Now it's running at fives and sixes and sometimes fours and fives ... We have generally five staff on in the morning and that's including a four-bedded coronary care unit.[4] There's never any more than one nurse in there. And that's including the person in charge.

SP   And this has a major effect on attempts to introduce new ...

SN(F)   It certainly does because all the time, you're fighting against time. We have 24 beds in this ward and constantly we are transferring patients out to other wards to bring new patients in. We are constantly full. In doing that we are increasing our workload as well, with the paperwork to transfer these people out, and they're probably our patients who are up and about and self-caring, and probably the ones we don't have to deal so much with, to bring in more acute patients all the time ... We also have patients on the ward awaiting surgery - bypass, valvular surgery, who need a lot of psychological care. We don't seem to have the time to sit down, discuss things, rediscuss things with them .. I feel they sometimes get pushed a bit to the side because we're bringing in these acute ones.

The problems associated with cutbacks in nursing salary budgets are not confined to extra pressure upon qualified staff. Correlating with a reduction of their numbers is a dramatic rise in the numbers of unqualified staff and a resultant alteration in the skill-mix balance. For example, in a single year from 1990 to 1991, the number of qualified nurses employed by the NHS fell by over 5 per cent, while the number of unqualified staff employed rose by 17 per cent (Ranade 1994).

This development in the profile of the nursing workforce once again reflects post-Fordist imperatives (Nettleton 1995). It is argued that a dual labour market consisting of a core of highly skilled workers and a periphery of more casual labour facilitates flexibility, in that the former group are flexible in terms of their skills, and the latter group in terms of their time. While such an arrangement may be of benefit to those lucky enough to be included in the core, the casualisation and marginalisation of employment for those on the periphery leads to low wages, insecure contracts and poor working conditions (Atkinson 1986). Moreover, despite the rhetoric of appropriate skill-mixes, there is evidence to suggest that there is a positive correlation between the standards of nursing care and the qualifications and training of nursing staff conducting that care (Carr-Hill 1992).

Conclusion

The effects of changes in state welfare provisions as a consequence of capitalist restructuring have been a double-edged sword as far as nurses are concerned. On the one hand, the development of flexible forms of production and consumption has tended to strengthen the relative status of nursing. On the other hand, the retrenchment of welfare state funding has put pressure on the nursing workforce, in many cases restricting their ability to operate nursing care above a very basic level of patient servicing. With increasing reliance on unqualified staff to perform the bulk of practical care, this problem is likely to be exacerbated in the future.

Notes

1. Flowline assembly entails the product flowing past the assembly worker, who works in one place. Dedicated machinery is purpose-built for each model of the product that is being produced.
2. McKinlay and Arches define proletarianisation as:

    > the process by which an occupational category is divested of control over certain prerogatives relating to the location, content and essentiality of its task activities and is thereby subordinated to the broader requirements of production under advanced capitalism (1985:161).

3. The first number refers to the nurses on duty during the morning, the second to the nurses on in the afternoon, which is higher because of the overlap of early and late shifts.
4. The morning shift is the busiest period of the nursing day.

9 Sub-structural influences

Introduction

The previous three chapters have discussed how various social structural processes affect the nature of nurse-doctor relations. The broad theoretical basis for these discussions was Bhaskar's critical realism. The basic assumptions of this position are that society, which pre-exists individuals, provides the necessary conditions for intentional human activity. It 'is an ensemble of structures, practices and conventions' (1989a:76) which provide actors with the stock of skills and competencies appropriate to their social contexts through the process of socialisation. However, this ensemble is not independent of human activity. It only continues to exist in any given form if individuals reproduce it through their intentional actions; the possibility of transformative human action means that it can be altered.

Like many other sociological models, Bhaskar concentrates his analysis on two levels - the societal and the individual, which are linked by socialisation in one direction and reproduction or transformation in the other (1989b). What I wish to suggest here is that the dyadic nature of this model glosses over the complexities of social relationships and situations. As Hannan observes:

> Available sociological theories do not appear to be capable of dealing successfully with more than two (partly nested) levels of analysis. Most theory and research on macrostructures elides distinctions between levels, tacitly converting multilevel processes into two-level ones. Most commonly, the problem is reduced to one involving persons and macrostructures (1992:121-2).

This may be rather too sweeping a judgement, in that there are theorists that have attempted to construct models that reflect multilevel processes.[1] Indeed, Bhaskar himself has recently argued that attention should be given to the 'gradation between degrees of distraction and licenses, within a unified concept of ontology, distinctions between global, regional, domain-specific and local ontologies' (1993:107). The purpose of this chapter is to do just that, thereby going beyond the over-simplified (but heuristically valuable) model of social\invididual dualism. It will be my contention that the Procrustean bed of binary analysis obscures the fact that the nurse-doctor relationship is affected by factors which emanate from a number of different levels of social organisation.

At least five different (but 'nested')[2] levels can be identified. Working from the macro to the micro level, these can be termed:

1. Social structural

2. Occupational

3. Organisational

4. Situational

5. Individual

By organising the analysis of nurse-doctor relations according to these five levels of analysis, I hope to highlight the complexity of social interaction.

The social structural level

Reflecting the shape of Bhaskar's model, this level of analysis is the one that I have largely concentrated on in the previous three chapters. The aim of these chapters was to examine how the social structural factors of gender, 'race' and economic relations affect the position of nurses and their interaction with doctors.

As I have indicated, these factors do not operate in isolation to each other. One mechanism may either reinforce or attenuate the effects of another. Thus, for example, the relationship between a white female nurse and a black male doctor involves the influence of two contradictory mechanisms. Patriarchal gender relations would tend to disempower the nurse, while racism would tend to disempower the doctor. Conversely, a male doctor's gendered position in relation to female nurses is reinforced by medicine's privileged position within capitalist relations of production.

Given that social situations are open systems, the actual effects of combinations of mechanisms can only be adduced through empirical examination.

Changes in social structures

To complicate matters further, the nature and effects of social structures are not immutable. While they may predate individual actors, they depend on those actors to reproduce them. Actors also have (limited) power to transform social structures.

In connection with gender relations, the effects of feminist attempts at transformation were seen in the increasing assertiveness of female nurses in their relations with male co-workers. As an archetypal female occupation, nursing's position over time reflects the changing position of women in general society.

At a more immediate level, the effects of racism were directly modified by some of the actors observed. Black doctors made use of their superior occupational position and formal knowledge to attenuate the deleterious consequences of the 'race' relations that pertained. The ability of Black doctors to reduce the influence of racism in their interactions with white nurses was based upon the ideology of professionalism which imbued the culture of both occupations.

The occupational level

This level of analysis pertains both to occupational culture and to the more or less formally defined remit of nursing and medicine. The aim of the section is to examine how these factors impinge upon power relations. Concerning culture, three aspects are discussed here. First, the professional culture that influences both occupations is addressed. Specifically, I examine nurses' beliefs about what they see as the appropriate division of labour between themselves and doctors. Second, I examine the culture of superiority that is specific to doctors. Third, the role that tradition plays in nursing deference is discussed. In relation to formal remits, I discuss differences in legal status and formal occupational knowledge.

Culture and occupational position

In examining how professional culture attenuated the effects of racism in Chapter Seven, I accorded professionalism a rather ambiguous structural existence. Here, I wish to underline the specific nature of professionalism. It differs from the other structural mechanisms that I identified in that, rather than enjoying a general social influence, it is specific to certain occupational groups. While patriarchy, racism and capitalism are systemic structures within the society examined, professionalism might be more accurately described as a sub-systemic structure. Indeed, using Parsonian theory, it could be further reduced to being a specific component of the cultural subsystem.

According to Parsons's (1951) typology of the social system, the cultural subsystem is one of its four basic components. The function of culture is to maintain the equilibrium of that system. He argues that it can do this because it consists of shared beliefs, interests and ideologies (Jenks 1993).

Nurses and doctors share many beliefs about the appropriate functions of, and relationship between, their respective occupations. The division of labour that pertains is often seen as being founded upon legal distinctions, the rationale for which lies in the clear requirements of professional service.

Transcript 9\1
Medical Ward

SP   How much influence do you think something like gender has over the nature of the occupational roles of doctors and nurses?

SN(F) I think you've been in sociology too long. Basically, I think those things don't matter too much at all. They and we have our jobs cut out for us. It is up to them to do certain things and us to do certain things. That's because we are in different professions, not different genders. Each profession has its own tasks. That's down to the law and not gender, or any of that sociology stuff. It's really simpler than you think. A doctor does what a doctor does because that's what his job is. I suppose I should say her as well, the sex thing doesn't matter, in terms of our professional roles anyway.

SP   Does it matter in other ways?

SN(F) Yes, I suppose it does. You get some doctors who think women are inferior and then they treat us worse than others. But that isn't to do with professional roles. What a doctor thinks or not of women doesn't have anything to do with the fact that only they can admit, only they can prescribe. Those are professional roles. They are rules laid down so that everyone knows their responsibility and their accountability. It would be total chaos if they weren't there.

SP   So, are these laid down in tablets of stone?

SN(F) No, no, of course not. Over time the professional role of the nurse has been changing, you know, the extended role and all that. But, the rules may change according to changed circumstances, but at any one time, you know what the rules are.

This might be seen as an example of what Bhaskar terms the unintentional reproduction of social structures:

People, in their conscious human activity, for the most part unconsciously reproduce (or occasionally, transform) the structures that govern their substantive activities of production. Thus people do not marry to reproduce the nuclear family, or work to reproduce the capitalist economy. But it is nevertheless the unintended consequence (and inexorable result) of, as it is also the necessary condition for, their activity (1989a:80).

Thus, the intentional actions of nurses and doctors vis-a-vis their division of labour, unintentionally reproduce (or on occasion, transform) social relations that are grounded in the structures of patriarchy, racism and capitalism. This occurs because the culture of professionalism provides the ideological support for the various formal aspects of the two occupations. These formal aspects will be discussed below.

To return to Parsons, it is now a sociological truism that his theoretical vision was flawed by a blindness to conflict. His portrayal of the cultural subsystem is no exception. We cannot assume that all those who share a cultural outlook will benefit equally from the material arrangements which that outlook justifies. Specifically, because nurses and doctors happen to share occupational beliefs and ideologies, we should not assume that they also share an identity of interest. On this point it might be more appropriate to turn to Marx: 'The ideas of the ruling class are in every epoch the ruling ideas' (1970:64). Thus it could be argued that the occupational culture provides the rationale for a formal system that is constructed to the advantage of the most powerful health care occupation, namely medicine. This advantage is reinforced by other aspects of occupational culture, namely doctors' belief in their own superiority, and nurses' continued reliance on tradition.

The medical culture of superiority

A significant facet of the occupational culture of doctors is the assumption of many that they are superior to nurses. While this ideology is more strongly expressed within the higher echelons of medicine, junior doctors are not immune from its effects. The statement of a Junior Medical Officer recounted in Chapter Six will be remembered:

Transcript 9\2
Metropolitan Hospital Medical Unit

JHO(M) Anyone can do a nurse's job, but there's not many people that can do what I can do.

However, we should be wary of assuming a general culture of superiority among doctors. There is some evidence to suggest that this sort of pompous ideology had less currency with female doctors.

Examination of medical students working in the ICU supports this thesis. The medical studies curriculum in the university attached to the hospital included the requirement that second year medical students should spend a week in hospital working in the capacity of nursing auxiliary. During my time of participant observation, two pairs of students, one pair female and one pair male, spent a week in the ICU. The attitudes of the two pairs to nursing were starkly different. While the female students took to the role of nursing auxiliary with gusto, the men indicated their level of commitment by arriving late, leaving early, and contriving to do as little as possible in the intervening period. One of them explained their dismissive attitude to this part of their course:

Transcript 9\3
Intensive Care Unit

MS(M)   We're only here for a week, and we're not going to be examined on it anyway. Sure, we're going to be doctors not nurses. The whole thing's pointless ... What sort of a training do you need to make a bed or empty a bedpan? If you ask me, its a week wasted which we could have spent learning something important.

The contrast in attitude between female and male medical students seen here shows just how deeply medical occupational culture is nested in the structured gender relations.

The male arrogance of these two very young health care workers caused considerable irritation among some nurses, who were not afraid to voice their misgivings. The student cited above was given a stark warning about the behaviour expected of him when he eventually qualified:

Transcript 9\4
Intensive Care Unit

EN(F)   If you want us to co-operate with you, you have to co-operate with us. Treat us properly if you want things done, if you don't want phone calls at four in the morning.

This transcript provides evidence that some nurses were no longer prepared to put up with the medical culture of superiority. What is more, we can see that they were well aware of the sanctions and weapons available to them in their efforts to counterbalance medical power.

However, by way of qualification, it should be noted that the culture of professionalism, with its emphasis on the value of functional specificity, encourages nurses to accept medicine as more intellectually demanding, and therefore more deserving of reward in both pecuniary and status terms. Melia (1987) observed in her study of student nursing culture that students valorised work associated with medicine, and denigrated work associated solely with nursing care activities, which they thought anyone could do, much in the same way as the JHO in Transcript 9\2. One nurse in this study was quite clear in her acceptance of functional stratification (cf. Davis and Moore 1945):

Transcript 9\5
Surgical Ward

SP   Do you think it's fair that he [consultant surgeon] gets what he gets, compared to you?

SN(F)   The long and the short of it is I couldn't do the things he does, and anyway, I wouldn't want the responsibility. You imagine the responsibility of opening someone up with a knife. Fair enough, I don't think nurses get paid enough, but I don't see we could make the case for getting as much as surgeons.

SP   What about status, the status that surgeons have compared to nurses?

SN(F)   No, I think to a good extent they earn their status. I don't think we have enough, but that isn't their fault.

However, the acceptance of the status of surgeons by this nurse did not extend to her happily acquiescing to their superior demeanour:

SP   So you think that [consultant surgeon] is justified in the way he acts towards nurses? That he deserves to act in that way because of his status?[3]

SN(F)   That's not what I am saying at all. That's a completely different matter. Just because of what he is shouldn't mean he gets away with treating us like dirt. Well, that's not really fair, he isn't really that bad except his off days.

SP   But do you not think that the superior manner goes with the status?

SN(F)   Hmmm Not necessarily. It depends on the person. With [new consultant surgeon], he gets the respect from nurses, but he doesn't rub our noses in it.

Notwithstanding the fact that many nurses appear to be happy with the fundamentals of the medical division of labour, we should remember that the nature of that division has shifted over time in nurses' favour. Section Two provided evidence that the historical subservience of nurses has been considerably attenuated over the last quarter of a century. We need to distinguish between acceptance of functional specificity and acceptance of the more extreme aspects of the medical culture of superiority.

Tradition

Transcript 9\5 provides an important qualification to the assumption that all things are in a state of flux. We need to be aware of the inertial power of tradition. Once patterns of behaviour become habitualised and institutionalised, it takes more than rationalist rejection to eradicate them. Ways of doing things that crystallised during the era of unmitigated nursing subservience continue to exert pressure over contemporary nurses (Dingwall and McIntosh 1978).

Nurses in the Intensive Care Unit were not infrequently observed to adopt the traditional handmaiden's role. An example of this occurred in an incident where a sister attempted to prevent a doctor from cleaning up the debris consequent to the insertion of an central venous cannula:

Transcript 9\6
Intensive Care Unit

SR(F)   [Enters room, sidles up to the doctor who has started to tidy away her debris, and gently tries to push her away from the trolley] Sure, leave that. We'll clear that stuff away for you. [Throws a sharp glance at the male SN (me) already in the room, and who had not offered to clear away the doctor's debris].

SHO(F) No, don't worry. I've still got gloves on, in case there are any nasties.

SR(F)   It's OK, I'll do it.

SHO(F) No really, I don't mind.

SR(F)   [Steps back and makes quizzical grimace at SN and leaves the room without a word.]

Yet again, we can see the pertinence of gender in this situation. First, it is hardly coincidental that it was a female doctor which insisted on tidying up (see discussion of frequency of tidying up by sex in Chapter Six). Secondly, it may not have been a coincidence that it was a male nurse who stood back and let her!

The situation recounted here is unusual in one respect, in that traditional, subservient actions performed by nurses in the ICU usually occurred in interactions between junior nursing and senior medical staff. This was especially noticeable in the context of the consultants' rounds, where it was the nurses' duty to push around the notes trolley and to select for the consultant the appropriate medical notes at each bedside, as well as to draw the curtains around each patient. While not all nurses tolerated such subservience, those who refused to comply with tradition, while they were tolerated, were seen as being deliberately heterodox, and were made aware by consultants that they were regarded as 'awkward'.

The inertia of tradition does not exclusively affect those nurses with recidivistic tendencies. On several occasions when I questioned nurses about their motivation for performing acts that appeared to me to be gratuitously demeaning, the nurses agreed with me in my evaluation, but explained their actions in terms of tradition. Consider the following example: A nurse was recording the frequency of a ventilated patient's respirations. This procedure required that she observe the patient and ventilator continuously for a minute. In the middle of this procedure, a consultant arrived at the bedside of an adjacent patient whose nurse was in the clinical room at the time. The consultant beckoned to the nurse at the next bed with the slightest nod of the head. She immediately desisted from her task in order to pull the curtains around the patient for the consultant. This was all he required of her. She stood behind the curtains with him in silence while he performed his examination. When he had finished, she redrew the curtains, and returned to restart her respirations observations all over again. She explained her actions to me by stating:

Transcript 9\7
Intensive Care Unit

SN(F)   Well, nurses have always been doing it, and it's a bit hard to stop now. I know I shouldn't have to do it but if I didn't he would have probably thrown the sheets back in front of everybody.

Again we return to the issue of patriarchy. There appears to have been two interconnected dynamics at play in this situation, both relating to what Hochschild (1983) terms emotional labour.

The first issue concerns what Hochschild calls the womanly art of status enhancement. She argues that part of women's role in patriarchal society is to emotionally service men through constant acts of deference. This deference has been formalised and commercialised in female-dominated service industries. Nurses are expected to cosset male colleagues in a subservient fashion. Because consultants' status expectations are so great, the pressure to pamper their egos is considerable.

Secondly, while the emotional servicing of male colleagues may be an implicit subtext of nurses' occupational lives, emotional labour in terms of caring for patients is their central explicit role (Smith 1992). The nurse in this instance felt an obligation to care for the patient who was approached by the consultant. She explained her action in terms of maintaining his emotional well-being by preventing his exposure and embarrassment. This sense of care towards the patient, combined with her perception that the consultant did not have the same sense of care, meant that she felt obliged to act in a subordinate fashion.

That it was the female nurse rather than the male doctor who was worried about the emotional well-being of the patient is hardly an accident. As James (1992) states, emotional labour is subject to gender division. Whether the importance of emotional labour to women is a contingent result of the fact that they have less access to power and status in patriarchal society, and therefore concentrate their efforts on making a resource out of feeling (Cline and Spender 1987), or whether it emerges from a fundamental sexual division in moral development (Gilligan 1982) is a thorny question that I will not pursue here. The point to be made is that women's caring is used (abused) in order to bolster male dominance; nurses' caring is used by doctors to bolster medical dominance.

It can be seen that, while some behaviour can be explained in terms of habit or tradition, such a level of analysis is not sufficient. We also need to ask what sorts of structural dynamics have shaped tradition. In this case, it has been seen that traditional nurse-doctors relations are largely predicated upon mechanisms resultant from the structure of patriarchy.

In addition to culture, there are more formal aspects of the occupations of nursing and medicine that have a powerful influence upon the power relations that pertain. Not least of these is the legal status that medicine enjoys.

Consideration of the legal system demonstrates a significant lacuna that results from the binary nature of critical realism. Bhaskar (1989a) argues that one of the fundamental factors distinguishing agents from structures is that only the former possesses intentionality. In the case of laws, while they affect most actors in an anonymous fashion, similar to the way social structures impinge upon individual reality, they are at the same time the creation of individuals who intended certain results from their legislative products. Now, it may be that the consequences of laws are often unintended; nevertheless, it remains the case that the sharp distinction between structure and agency that Bhaskar insists upon sits ill with the combined intentional human creation and structural effects of laws.

One way of conceiving the production of legislation is to categorise it terms of the actions of what Mouzelis (1991) terms macro actors. He argues that the actions of people in privileged positions in the social hierarchy, because they contribute unequally to the construction of social reality, cannot be limited to the 'micro level' of analysis.

The British legal system endows doctors with many powers. They have control over admission and discharge. They also have a near monopoly over diagnosis and prescription.[4] Perhaps most surprising, given the increasing popularity of the ethos of openness of care, doctors still enjoy almost absolute legal control over the amount of information that patients should be given about their illness, prognosis or treatment. Doctors' power in this area extends to being able to prevent nurses from communicating with patients if they feel that the knowledge communicated would be detrimental to the patient's health (Young 1994).

The fact that so many of the functions of doctors are set in the historical cement of legal statute has the effect of slowing down any momentum towards change.

Transcript 9\8
Nursing Development Unit

SN(F) We have come a long way, but at the end of the day, you can only go so far. There are things that it is simply not legal for us to do. Maybe we are taking most of the decisions in discharge, or admission, or whatever, but at the end of the day, because it is them [doctors] that has to sign on the dotted line, that gives them power.

In the other units examined, medical monopolies were in far wider active use than they were in the Nursing Development Unit. This was especially noticeable in the Intensive Care Unit, where, upon entry, patients were immediately subject to a medical examination, after which the medical officer made a provisional diagnosis, which stood until subsequent clinical evidence, or the opinion of a senior colleague contradicted it. This procedure was performed in a solitary fashion, behind closed curtains. This meant that the nurse had virtually no opportunity to influence the process. Thus the absolute control of doctors over diagnosis and prescription was, in this situation, not only *de jure*, but also *de facto*.

A number of the nurses from units in Suburban Hospital other than the Nursing Development Unit intimated that the only time when they encroached upon a clearly demarked line of acceptable diagnostic remit was when the unexpected occurred. Several used the example of cardiac arrest, where, because of the importance of swift intervention, nurses with sufficient training were allowed to diagnose the condition, and to prescribe and administer electrical defibrillation if they saw fit.

Because of the level of observation and control over patients in the ICU, the unexpected rarely occurred. In addition, even when something remiss did happen, there was always a physician at hand in the unit. As a consequence, nurses had no significant opportunity for any involvement in diagnosis. Even areas that were traditionally within the nursing remit, such as fluid intake and pressure area care, were closely supervised by medical staff.

Formal occupational knowledge

The legal status of doctors is bestowed upon them by dint of the credentials they gain through successful attainment of occupational qualifications. It is by these credentials that their occupational monopoly is maintained. It will be remembered that in Chapter Four I discussed the relationship between credentialism and social closure. At this point I wish to draw attention to the related issue of the formal occupational knowledge that provides the basis for the qualifications attained by doctors, and, indeed, for the culture of superiority that many of them are imbued with.

Empirical data from all the units examined indicated that there was little doubt that the formal biological knowledge possessed by medical staff was considerably greater than that of even the best qualified nurses. The most striking example of this was cited in the discussion on racism, where the African clinical expert in the ICU quite deliberately demonstrated the ignorance of nurses by showing up their inability to identify evidence of pulmonary surgery from a chest X-ray.

The lack of knowledge possessed by nurses meant that, in many instances, they were simply incapable of making decisions, even if they had wanted to. Doctors' control over diagnosis was thus strongly reinforced by their superior knowledge base.

The differential in formal knowledge was freely admitted by nurses, and was seen as a fundamental factor in determining the division of labour between the two occupations:

Transcript 9\9
Surgical Ward

SN(F)   When it comes down to it, we are trained to do different things. More to the point they are trained to do, to know, far more things. They go to university and learn all about the workings of the body for five years. Our training is only three, and even at that, most of it was spent as a dog's body on the ward, which doesn't give you all that much theoretical knowledge. A lot of the difference in our work, when it comes down to it, is due to the stuff they know and the stuff we don't know.

There are signs, however, that the gulf between nurses' and doctors' knowledge about health and illness may be narrowing. A number of the nurses interviewed identified Project 2000 (P2K) training, with its emphasis on academic work, as a conduit for change:

Transcript 9\10
Surgical Ward

SN(F)   I think things may well change over the next few years, when nurses trained through P2K actually start taking up staffing posts. You can see it already in the P2K students that we've had on the ward. They know a lot more than we did when we were at that stage, and what's more, they are not afraid to show it. I don't think doctors will be able to get away with the 'I know best' line that they use to put us in our place with the P2K ones. I think they will have to think and justify themselves and the actions they decide on a lot more.

Nurses' interest in theoretically founded practice is not restricted to those being trained through Project 2000. That nursing must be predicated upon intellectual activity is an assumption that has filtered its way into the attitudes of almost all nurses. However, because it poses a threat to the medical culture of superiority, the increasing knowledge of nurses has not been universally accepted with equanimity by their medical colleagues. More traditional doctors especially, do not take kindly to nurses attempting to alter care regimes on the grounds of the nurses' research-based knowledge. This, not unnaturally, leads to frustration on the part of nurses, as the account of this experienced staff nurse demonstrates:

Transcript 9\11
Surgical Ward

SN(F)   I think that some of the doctors have resented the fact that nurses now are making decisions and bringing their own points of view, because we have done research into things and are bringing points that some of

170

the doctors would not have known. I'll give you an example. This clamping and releasing of catheters. I, many many years ago, suggested that the big thing with a catheter was to ensure free drainage and why clamp it because you are not allowing free drainage and you are allowing the urine to be static? Nobody would listen to me. There was no point at that stage a nurse making a suggestion - nobody listened to you. Well then there was research done by nurses that proved that this clamping and releasing of catheters was no good, that you would be better explaining to the patient 'Look, you have a catheter in now. Maybe every hour, feel as if you are going to pass water and then hold back for a second and let go with the catheter in to continue bladder drill' Mind you, a lot of the doctors still say that's not much cop but it has all been proved. [Recently retired consultant] would not hear of it - we still had to clamp and release the catheters and a nurse in this hospital who had a degree brought it forward to him - they tried very hard, they brought in the research but he didn't want to know, but that has changed now. With the [contemporary surgeon], you can go ahead, but the older men will not change.

This transcript provides a good example of how the medical culture of superiority can be breached by nurses through the co-option of the grounds upon which that culture is founded, namely the possession of rational scientific knowledge. However, the brute occupational power that doctors still enjoy means that consultants like the one above are able to stand firm in the face of such an assault on their authority. Nevertheless, the transcript also indicates that this sort of recalcitrance may be becoming less of an option, even for consultant surgeons.

The nurse cited above was not the only one to identify the fact that consultants (especially older ones) were least likely to accredit nurses as possessing valid knowledge. Junior doctors, perhaps less self-confident about their own knowledge and occupational superiority, tended to be less dismissive:

Transcript 9\12
Surgical Ward

SP   Have you noticed if the new roles have changed the way you deal with doctors, for example?

SN(F)   I don't really know. I always found that if you passed on information, or gave your opinion, most of the JHOs would usually listen to you anyway, you know, take part of your advice or guidance on decision making. Some obviously wouldn't, but they only know a limited amount themselves. When they come out, it is putting all their theory into practice really. You have sort of seen the things and done the things before.

171

SP   Given you qualified only three and a half years ago, you would have been coming out with all the New Nursing roles. What you are saying is that you never felt any problem asserting your opinions to ...

SN(F)   Not with the JHOs. Sometimes, the consultants - that would be a totally different situation because they don't really want to listen very much to you. It's much more obvious with them. I mean, you wouldn't have the same relationship with the consultant as you would with your JHO. The SHOs, usually, most of them would take into account what you are saying.

SP   Expand a bit on the consultants.

SN(F)   They listen to the information you're giving, but, you might have one view of what the patient might need or want, and you voice your opinion, but the consultant has got his own idea and, regardless really of what you are saying, at the end of the day, he's going to stick to his decision, I think. Whereas you could discuss a situation better with your JHO or SHO and maybe come to a compromise.

It is no coincidence that the above transcripts were all from statements made by nurses working in surgery. Consultant surgeons have a notorious reputation amongst nurses for being the most arrogant breed of doctor.

The organisational level

This level refers to the effects that specific organisational structures within which nurses worked, had upon their occupational position. Specifically, it examines how unit organisation affects the degree to which nurses have extended their clinical role.

The extended role of the nurse

Over the past few years there has been a selective extension of the role of the nurse. The major driving force behind this development was the policy decision to reduce the hours worked by junior doctors. Because recruitment of doctors did not increase at a rate commensurate with the decrease in time that each doctor worked, many health care institutions looked to nurses to fill the gap by encouraging them to perform some tasks that were previously done by doctors. These tasks included performing phlebotomies, and the administration of intravenous drugs and fluids and of blood transfusions. Nurses were usually required to attain a certificate of competence before they were allowed to perform such tasks.

During the period of data gathering, whether or not nurses were asked to perform such tasks was at the discretion of the specific health care institutions. Indeed, even

172

within one hospital, nurses on different units were authorised to carry out different extended roles. Because this variance was the result of organisational factors, discussion of the extended role is located in this section.

The nurse's role had been most extended in the intensive care unit. Nurses in the unit were able to perform tasks, such as the administration of intravenous drugs, which few other nurses in that hospital were allowed to do.

Their extended role was a source of pride for many of the nurses in the intensive care unit. I gained the impression that they felt that being entrusted with tasks that other nurses were not permitted to perform set them apart from the mass. An example of this sort of attitude was implied in my welcome from one of the unit's sisters:

Transcript 9\13
Intensive Care Unit

SR(F)   Have you ever worked in an intensive care unit before?

SP   No, apart from a couple of days observing during training, this is my
          first time.

SR(F)   Well, don't worry if you find it a bit daunting at first. There will be a
          lot of things we do here that are not done on other units, so don't worry
          if you are unsure of anything. If you are unsure, just ask one of the
          staff. They won't mind because we all realise that being in intensive
          care is different, and that there are things that you wouldn't have learnt
          to do on the wards. By the time you go back to university you will be
          able to do a lot of things that you didn't have experience of either as a
          student or a staff nurse.

Ironically, while their extended role may have gained the intensive care nurses a degree of kudos, it did nothing to empower them in their relations with doctors; in fact, the opposite was the case. Because their extended roles were by nature paramedical, they remained under the close control of doctors. Thus, while ICU nurses had the authority to administer intravenous drugs, they did not have the authority to decide which drugs should be given, which doses they should be given in, or when they should be given. In effect, their extended roles tied these nurses even closer in their subservient relationship with medical colleagues. Their gain in status was more than matched by their loss of power.

Not all nurses were seduced by the kudos of the extended role. Indeed, some were forcefully antipathetic to it:

Transcript 9\14
Medical Ward

SP   What are your views on the extended role of the nurse?

SN(F)   I think, well, I think it's a load of crap, really, if you'll excuse my language. All you are doing is JHO's dirty work. It's not nursing work, so
why should nurses have to do it? We have quite enough to do as it is.

This sort of antipathy is far from exceptional. The extended role has been
contrasted (often unfavourably) with what has been termed the expanded role of the
nurse, which refers to those areas clearly within the remit of nursing that have
developed over recent years:

Some nurses would argue that extending their role to take on jobs that doctors
might wish to delegate is of a different order to an expanded role. The latter is
much more in line with the nursing responsibilities advanced by the proponents
of the 'New Nursing' (Robinson *et al.* 1992:60).

This argument entails the assumption that innovations like primary nursing and
patient advocacy provide a preferred route for the development of the occupation.
However, it is possible to argue that the extended and expanded roles are not
necessarily mutually opposing. This thesis was put to me by the ward sister of the
surgical ward:

Transcript 9\15
Surgical Ward

SR(F)   There is also the reduction of doctors' hours, therefore we are being
asked to take on extended roles as it were. Having said that, there are a
few courses that some of us have been on, but our perception of why we
are doing this, I think is different. For example, I can speak personally
about the IV additive certificate. Now it was seen when we first started
the course by the consultant who came to speak to us that we would be
doing this in order to help in the reduction in doctors' hours. We were
there, however, under a different premise insofar as we felt that we
were there to take on this role to add a more holistic approach for
patient care, and that was really the only reason that we felt we wanted
to do it. Obviously, we went ahead and finished the course, but I still
think the two ideas are not in agreement as to why we were actually
doing it.

SP   When I was working in ICU, I noticed that ICU nurses were proud of
the fact that while ward nurses were not able to do these things, that
they were. But it didn't actually make any difference. They were almost
more supervised by the medical staff because they were doing
paramedical jobs all the time.

SR(F)   I would be very concerned that we wouldn't take on this role to the detriment of other nursing care that should be done. We are taking this on over and above what we would normally do and if at the end of the day other things were suffering, patient care was suffering for that, then I would obviously have to question that.[5] But again, it does give a more holistic approach to patient care, and I think we are best placed to do that sort of thing. And, let's face it, our techniques probably would be a lot better. I don't know whether I should be saying this or not, but it is a proven fact that our techniques would be a lot safer.

The argument made by this sister, that if they are to be of any benefit to nursing care, extended roles need to be co-opted into a holistic framework, is one that has gained official acceptance. Indeed, the UKCC has gone even further by attacking the grounds on which the extended role has been constructed:

The practice of nursing has traditionally been based on the premise that pre-registration education equips the nurse to perform at a certain level and to encompass a particular range of activities. It is also based on the premise that any widening of that range and enhancement of the nurse's practice requires 'official' extension of that role by certification.

The Council considers that the terms 'extended' or 'extending' roles which have been associated with this system are no longer suitable since they limit, rather than extend, the parameters of practice. As a result, many practitioners have been prevented from fulfilling their potential for the benefit of patients. The Council also believes that concentration on 'activities' can detract from the importance of holistic nursing care ...

... **In order to bring into proper focus the professional responsibility and consequent accountability of individual practitioners, it is the Council's principles for practice rather than certificates for tasks which should form the basis for adjustments to the scope of practice** (UKCC 1992a:7-8, emphasis in original).

The change in policy that this position statement implied was not optional:

This change has consequences for managers of clinical practice and professional leaders of nursing, ... who must ensure that local policies and procedures are based upon the principles set out in this paper (UKCC 1992a:13).

It appears that the UKCC has recognised that the extended role, with its implications of medical gatekeeping and supervision, compromises the autonomy of nurses, and its response can be seen as an assertion of the nurse's right to professional autonomy. The central thrust of the *Scope of Professional Practice* position statement is that nurses themselves, using the guidelines formulated by the UKCC, should be allowed to use their own professional judgement to decide which roles are appropriate for them to adopt.

Unfortunately, in terms of the empirical data collected for this book, the practical ramifications of the UKCC's position had yet to impinge upon nursing practice. However, the data do show that the strategy adopted by their statutory body was in consonance with many nurses' feelings on the issue.

The situational level

In this section, I wish to return to David Hughes's paper on nurse-doctor interaction. Hughes argued that the contention of his paper was that:

> to the extent that medical sociologists have accepted over-deterministic versions of [the professional dominance] thesis, they have underplayed the situated nature of medical control and of nurse deference ... This is not to say, of course, that the expected relationship of 'medical dominance' breaks down completely, but that various work exigencies mean that its impact is considerably weakened in many informal interactions (1988:16).

Situational exigencies of work were also found in this study, two of which will be discussed below. First, I will discuss how night duty work allowed nurses greater latitude, and second, how nurses' informal occupational knowledge advantaged them in their dealings with doctors.

The freedom of night duty

The ramifications of night work for nurse-doctor relations are an example of how situational exigencies are nested in organisational frameworks. The working hours of nurses and doctors are organised on different lines. Doctors' working arrangements usually take two forms: as a rule they are present on duty from 9am to 5pm, Monday to Friday. Outside these hours, they take it in turns to be available on an 'on-call' basis. This means that, while they are not present on the wards, they are available if the nurses on duty feel that they are required.[6] The more junior the doctor, the more on-call duty they are required to perform. Nurses, on the other hand, work according to a shift system, which means that there are always nurses on duty, whatever hour and whatever day. At nights and at weekends, therefore, nurses are on their own in the wards, and it is up to their discretion whether they feel it necessary to call for medical assistance. Thus, the organisation of working hours creates a situational exigency which allows nurses to take more responsibility for decision making at night than they otherwise enjoy.

In Chapter Five, I recounted an incident where a sister on night duty had discontinued a morphine pump during the night without prior medical permission. This trespass into the grounds of medical decision-making was met with equanimity on the part of the doctor whom she informed of her action in the morning, the reason being that she had saved the doctor from being woken in the middle of the night.

In order to test whether this was an isolated incident, or whether it was an example of a general pattern, I asked a staff nurse working on night duty on a medical unit in the same hospital to document the number of times that doctors were called onto the ward, and the reasons for which they were called, over a period of four nights. During this 40-hour period, the nurses on duty asked the doctor on call to come to the ward on only three occasions. All three call outs were in response to the arrival of a new patient (the admission of a new patient by a medical practitioner being a compulsory requirement). Apart from admissions, the night duty nurses relied entirely on themselves. The organisationally generated situational exigency of working on their own gave nurses considerable autonomy in their work.

Informal occupational knowledge

It will be remembered from the discussion on formal occupational knowledge that doctors' superior grasp of formal knowledge was one of the foundations of their superordinate occupational position. However, nurses were able to make up for some of this imbalance through their knowledge of specific procedures. This was clearly seen in the intensive care unit.

Because only registrars and above were involved in the unit for more than a few months at a time, there was a high turnover of medical staff. In contrast, some nurses had been working in the unit since it had opened over a decade previously. Nurses with experience of the unit had considerable advantage in their relationships with doctors who were inexperienced in the ways that things were run. In effect, the roles of knowledgeable doctor and ignorant nurse were reversed:

Transcript 9\16
Intensive Care Unit

SHO(M) [About to take a blood sample for blood cultures] Do I have to wear a gown?

EN(F)   No, I'll let you off with that. [Laughs]

SHO(M) Thank you very much you are very kind.

Despite the fact that this nurse had superior knowledge, she felt obliged to display the 'mandatory smile' (Cline and Spender 1987) of deference by turning the role reversal into a joke. Those nurses who fail to disguise their advantage are open to being stigmatised as domineering:

177

SP   What rate do you want this feed to go through?

SHO(F) Hmmm ... I suppose we should try him at 10 mils for the first hour and see if he tolerates it.

SP   Well, we tried him on milk yesterday and it was fine.

SHO(F) I'm not quite sure then ... What is the normal rate?

SP   I'm not sure, I think it might be 15 mils per hour.

SHO(F) I tell you what, we'll start it at 15 mils until Sister [Surname] arrives at lunch time. I'm sure she will be able to give us chapter and verse about how it's meant to be done. [Aside to another staff nurse] We'll leave it up to our little führer.

The fact that the SHO who denigrated the sister was female suggests a qualification to the discussion earlier in this chapter on the medical culture of superiority: while it may be largely a male phenomenon, it is not exclusively so.

The individual level

This exception to my argument that there was a connection between maleness and the medical culture of superiority is a reminder of the contingent nature of social reality. Bhaskar argues that 'the objects of social scientific enquiry ... only ever manifest themselves in open systems; that is, in systems where invariant empirical regularities do not obtain' (1989b:45). While social structures influence the manner in which individuals behave, they do not determine people's actions. To seek to identify invariant laws through the display of invariant actions is to misconstrue the possibilities of social knowledge.

I include the individual level here to stress the fact that, in my identification of generalities of behaviour, I am not making any universal claims. While I have identified many tendencies of behaviour and attitude resulting from the influence of social factors, these are no more than tendencies. At all levels of analysis, because of factors contingent to the persons involved, I found exceptions to the 'rules' that I was positing.

The occupational world is only one part of a person's life and history. There is a myriad of influences that go into the formation of a person's character. There is therefore a myriad of responses to the enablements and constraints of social structure. For example, explanation of the fact that some female junior nurses were extremely assertive in their dealings with doctors, while others were subservient, cannot be entirely framed in terms of different structural, occupational, organisational, or even situational positions. While explanation of the psychological factors that influence the ways that individuals act lies outside the sociological scope of this book, it is important to recognise their significance.

Conclusion

The purpose of this chapter has been to qualify the over-simplistic society\individual duality that animated the previous three chapters. By analysing nurse-doctor interactions at five different levels of analysis, the complex nature of social interaction has been highlighted. Indeed, even with the expansion to five levels of analysis, there was still a degree of arbitrary classification.

The levels of analysis should not be regarded as discrete; they are characterised by significant interpolation. This interpolation is not confined to the nesting of contiguous levels. In partial defence of Bhaskar's dualism, it should be noted that the effects of social structures impinge upon all the levels of social organisation identified here. Similarly, the reflexive nature of individuals will affect how they respond to the enablements and constraints entailed at all levels.

Notes

1. See, for example, Aldrich's (1992) proposal for a five-level model of analysis, which consists of community, populations, organisations, groups and individuals.
2. By nested I mean 'placed or fitted inside another, such that each item or constituent contains or is contained within another similar one in a hierarchical arrangement (New Shorter Oxford Dictionary).
3. At the start of the interview, we had been discussing the ways of this particular surgeon, whom I had also worked with when I was employed in Suburban Hospital.
4. By way of qualification, I should reiterate that, in relation to diagnosis, the nursing process, with its category of nursing diagnosis has had the effect of blurring the parameters of this medical monopoly. As far as prescription is concerned, nurses have recently made some inroads here as well. The *Medical Products: Prescriptions by Nurses Act*, 1992 has given suitable qualified community nurses the right to prescribe from a limited formulary.
5. The sister's concern here is very much in line with the concerns of the UKCC, whose *Scope of Professional Practice* document states:

> the registered nurse ... must ensure that any enlargement or adjustment of the scope of professional practice must be achieved without compromising or fragmenting existing aspects of professional practice and care (1992a:6).

6. The intensive care unit was a partial exception to this rule. There was always a senior house officer on the unit. However, while SHOs continued to be present during weekends and in the evenings, at night they slept in a room on the unit provided for that purpose, to be woken if and when the nurse in charge felt necessary.

10 Conclusion

Substantive conclusions

This chapter is divided into two sections. In the first section, I summarise the conclusions of my research, and in the second, I discuss their import. The substantive focus of this book was concentrated in Parts Two and Three; these will be addressed in turn.

Part Two

It will be remembered that Part Two dealt with the development of nurse-doctor relations. In Chapter Three I outlined the history of this relationship. I noted that there was evidence that in the 1920s and 1930s, nurses were in a position of unmitigated subordination to doctors. However, by the 1960s, the nature of nurse-doctor relations had changed. Stein (1978 [1966]) identified what he called the 'doctor-nurse game' as the dominant mode of interaction. This involved nurses having a surreptitious involvement in decision making processes.

Examination of the evidence subsequent to the original publication of Stein's paper indicated that the process of democratisation of inter-occupational relations has continued. Under the aegis of the nursing process, starting in North America in the 1970s, and spreading to Britain at the end of that decade, nursing began to challenge the monopoly of control over work that medicine had hitherto enjoyed. In addition, informal interactions between nurses as doctors noted by commentators such as Hughes (1988) displayed considerable assertiveness on the part of nurses.

This is not to say that the advancement of nursing was unproblematic. Many clinical nurses found the ideological aspirations of nursing entrepreneurs to be unrealistic, in that they were unable to overcome the material restraints of a health care system centred around medical dominance. However, by the late 1980s and early 1990s, most commentators were convinced that the occupational position of nursing *vis-à-vis* medicine had altered significantly in nursing's favour.

Chapter Four supplemented the account of the previous chapter by looking specifically at the strategies that nursing entrepreneurs used to advance their occupation. It was noted that these strategies took cognisance of the ideas emanating from the sociology of professions.

I divided the development of the sociology of professions into three distinct phases. The first phase entailed the dominance of trait and professionalisation approaches. Professionalisation theory, especially, has had a considerable impact upon the ideology of nursing entrepreneurs. The second phase involved the emergence of critical theories, in their neo-Weberian, Marxist, and radical guises. However, during the same period, a phenomenological perspective, which concentrated on the interpretations of professional actors was also developing. The third phase saw the introduction of feminism into the discourse on professions. The achievement of feminist occupational sociology was to bridge the dichotomy between critical and phenomenological approaches.

New Nursing entrepreneurs have taken this synthesis to heart. On the one hand, the phenomenological aspect means that the experiences and perspectives of nurses are valued. On the other hand, the application of critical approaches to established male professions have provided nursing with the theoretical tools to challenge medical dominance.

The use of the nursing process as an independent diagnostic and prescriptive system can be seen as an example of the dual closure strategy identified by neo-Weberians, in that it entails usurpation of previous medical monopolies, and exclusion, in that control over the process is restricted in Britain to 'first level' nurses. Nurses have also taken cognisance of radical theories. The New Nursing promotion of active patient participation in care can be seen as an implicit response to the assault on the power and privilege of established professions by radical theorists such as Illich (1981). However, while practical strategies have developed in response to recent sociological writings on the professions, the conception of professions promulgated by trait theorists continues to be used as ideological justification by some nursing entrepreneurs.

Chapter Five involved a description of contemporary nurse-doctor power relations using the empirical data that I gathered. This description was ordered according to four ideal types of interaction that emerged from examination of the historical literature. The first type was termed unmitigated subordination. This involved clear superordination on the part of doctors and subordination on the part of nurses. The second ideal type, which I called informal covert decision making, related to the playing of the doctor-nurse game noted by Stein. The third type, informal overt decision making, emerged from works such as that of Hughes (1988), who noted that nurses' influence in informal interactions was considerable. The final ideal type, formal overt decision making, corresponded to the new legal status of nursing diagnosis and prescription entailed in the adoption of the nursing process.

All four ideal typical modes of interaction were manifested in the research data. Sometimes, nurses acted in an unmitigatedly subordinate fashion, although occurrences of this type were rare, and usually involved exchanges between senior medical and junior nursing staff. These types of actors also occasionally played the doctor-nurse game. However, use of the game was far less than might be expected, given the assumptions of many commentators about its prevalence. However, while nurses are no longer expected to pretend an inability to make decisions, they are still expected by doctors to be deferential, and in cases of disagreement, to acquiesce to medical decisions.

However, notwithstanding medical expectations, nurses were frequently observed to make informal suggestions about care to doctors, and were on occasion prepared to stand their ground in the face of medical disagreement. Informal overt decision making was a widely practised nursing strategy, used with differing degrees of assertiveness, depending on the situation and the status of the nurse and doctor involved.

The capacity to make formal decisions about care had considerably less impact than informal strategies. It was noted that the nursing process was not used to organise care in the ICU, although process documentation was completed in order to satisfy medico-legal requirements. In Suburban Hospital, while the process was used to organise nursing care, it had limited impact upon the division of labour. The exception to this rule was the Nursing Development Unit, where the nursing process was incorporated into strategies of nursing empowerment.

The chapter concluded by noting that, while all four ideal types of interaction occurred, there was evidence that power relations between nurses and doctors had altered in favour of rational dialogue, at a cost to discourse based upon the unquestioned power of doctors. However, while nurses felt more able to make their voices heard, their position was still limited by the power that remained in the hands of their medical colleagues.

Part Three

Part Three examined the factors that affected nurse-doctor relations. In line with the tenets of critical realism, three of the chapters in this part were dedicated to the examination of the relationship between social structures and the interactions of nurses and doctors.

Chapter Six examined the crucial issue of gender relations. I argued that the occupational position of nursing was located within the structure of patriarchy. I looked first of all at how different gender permutations influenced the nature of nurse-doctor interactions. I noted that the sex of the nurse had little influence upon the quality of interactions, but the sex of the doctor did, with interactions between female doctors and nurses being more egalitarian. I concluded that the fact that nurses' gender had far less impact than doctors' indicated the power differential that still existed between the two groups overall. Being in a weaker occupation meant that nurses had less opportunity to engineer the quality of relationships with doctors, and as a consequence male nurses were unable to utilise the advantages that they gained from their gender.

Examination of nurses' attitudes to gender issues revealed that while nurses frequently objected in a vociferous fashion to assumptions by doctors about their inferior gendered roles, these objections were usually directed at discrete individuals. Nurses did not see medical dominance in toto as being structured by patriarchy. However, they were more prepared to utilise gendered explanations for the intra-occupational advantages enjoyed by male nurses. I explained this difference in terms of the persuasiveness of the credentialist claims of medicine; claims which male nurses had difficulty in making because female nurses had direct experience of sexist discrimination.

In examining sexual stereotyping, I found no evidence to support the popular image of nurses as being sexually promiscuous with medical colleagues. Unsurprisingly, nurses deeply resented being portrayed in such as fashion.

I found no evidence of sexual harassment of female nurses during participant observation in the Intensive care Unit. However, the interactions of this unit seemed to be somewhat of an exception, in that there was evidence from other units that it occurred, sometimes in very blatant forms.

Finally, I noted a confidence in nurses about their status as female workers. Contrary to previous studies, they did not valorise present or future domestic roles over their occupational aspirations.

The chapter concluded by noting that while gender remains a crucial factor in the occupational position of nursing, its effect appears to be changing over time. The rather convoluted nature of nurse-doctors relations appears to reflect gender relations at a societal level, which have involved a degree of female empowerment since the advent of second wave feminism. However, there is a need for caution, in that while patriarchal influence over relations between nurses and doctors may have been partially attenuated, within nursing itself the dominance of men continues to expand.

Chapter Seven focused on the social structure of racism. The discussion on racism was framed around Hughes's (1988) paper, in which he found that interactions between white nurses and Asian doctors often involved a breakdown of nurses' deference. This was not the case in my study. The explanation posited for this empirical divergence was that black and Asian doctors in my study were familiar with the linguistic and cultural mores of the country they were working in, while the doctors studied by Hughes were not. However, I argued that it would be misleading to extrapolate from this that breakdowns in nursing deference could be explained in purely functional terms. Backstage interactions between nurses demonstrated that some indulged in racist discourse. My explanation for simultaneous backstage racism and frontstage propriety was that the structure of racism was modified by the professional ideology to which nurses adhered. Because the doctors in my study could not be criticised on the grounds of competence, an important avenue for the frontstage expression of racism was cut off. I noted that at least one of the doctors in the study seemed to be aware of this, and deliberately set out to reinforce his reputation as a clinical expert in order to obviate racist denigration. This was seen as an example of how human agents are capable of transforming the effects of structures.

In relation to the question of why nurses adhered to professional ideology frontstage, but reverted to racism backstage, I adopted Bourdieu's (1990) theory of practice, and in particular his concept of habitus to argue that nurses live in both lay and occupational habiti, which contain contradictory assumptions.

Chapter Eight considered how the nature of capitalism affects inter-occupational relations within public health care institutions. I argued that doctors had traditionally enjoyed a privileged position within western economies, but that recent developments in capitalism had tended to undermine that privilege. I focused on two processes: the retrenchment of welfare state expenditure and the introduction of post-Fordist modes of production and consumption.

I argued that organisational reforms of health care, motivated by the desire to control costs, had an indirect effect upon nurse-doctor relations. Because they involved the decimation of nursing middle management, the Griffiths reforms entailed clinical nurses taking on more responsibility. This gave ward sisters the chance to have an input into strategic hospital decision making, and allowed more junior nurses to take more responsibility for clinical care. This meant that junior nurses were now dealing directly with doctors, rather than receiving medical orders that had been filtered down through the ward sister. Thus, extra administrative burdens had the effect of enhancing the influence of clinical nurses at all levels.

The move towards post-Fordist flexibility also benefited nurses. This was most clearly seen in the opening of a Nursing Development Unit which provided an alternative model of health care, one in which nurses were the central actors.

The chapter concluded with a note of caution. The increased nursing autonomy that resulted from managerial reforms and the introduction of alternative modes of care has been bought at the price of extra work, which often restricts opportunities for the introduction of New Nursing procedures. In addition, it has to be remembered that, as a result of health care rationalisation, increasing numbers of nurses are unemployed.

The final chapter in Part Three departed from the structure\action duality of critical realism in order to examine factors affecting nurse-doctor relations using a multi-level approach. Factors emanating from five different levels of social organisation were addressed.

The first level of analysis concentrated on social structures. I noted that structural factors do not operate in isolation to each other. Because they exist within an open social system, the effects of one may either attenuate or reinforce the effects of another. In addition, the nature and effects of structures depend upon actors to reproduce or transform them. As a consequence they are subject to change.

The next level to be addressed was the occupational level. Here I examined both occupational culture and the formally defined remits of medicine and nursing. In terms of culture, I noted that both nurses and doctors tended to accept the fundamentals of the division of labour which divided the occupations. This was reinforced by a culture of superiority on the part of doctors and a culture of tradition on the part of nurses. This was despite the fact that many nurses were resentful of doctors' presumptions of superiority, and, indeed, of their own rather unwilling adherence to tradition. Indeed, despite their acceptance of the validity of the division of labour that pertained between nursing and medicine, many nurses were unprepared to put up with expressions of superiority on the part of doctors.

Examination of more formal occupational characteristics showed that the legal status of doctors was a major factor in the maintenance of their occupational superordination. This was reinforced by their superior formal occupational knowledge, although there were signs that, with the advent of Project 2000 nurse training, the gap in formal occupational knowledge will narrow.

The third level to be examined was the organisational level. Here, I used the example of how unit organisation affected the degree to which nurses had extended their clinical role.

A correlation was noted between the technocentricity of a unit and the sort of tasks that nurses on the unit were allowed to perform. In highly technocentric units such as the ICU, nurses had adopted a number of paramedical roles. However, despite the kudos that this extension of role gave to nurses in the ICU, it did little for their occupational autonomy, in that paramedical tasks were closely supervised by doctors, while more basic nursing tasks were not.

The compromising of autonomy entailed in the extended role of the nurse has been recognised by the UKCC, who have decreed that it should be the responsibility of individual nursing practitioners to decide which roles they feel are appropriate for them to adopt.

The situational level referred to the effects of situational exigencies upon nurse-doctor relations. Two examples were used. First, it was noted that nurses on night duty, because there are no doctors present unless called by nurses, enjoy considerable autonomy over their work. Second, because nurses tend to be employed in specific units for longer periods of time than do doctors, they accumulate considerable informal knowledge about the workings of those units. The informal occupational knowledge of nurses goes some way to counterbalance the formal occupational knowledge of doctors.

The final level was the individual level. Because this is the subject of psychology, it was beyond the remit of this book. However, I argued that its importance should not be underestimated, in that some variations of behaviour could not be explained through examination of the other levels.

The significance to nursing

As I have noted previously, Bhaskar (1989a) argues that knowledge is a necessary, though insufficient requirement for freedom. One of the prime goals of this book is to elucidate the occupational position of nursing, and to identify

186

the constraints and enablements entailed in its social structural position. It is my hope that the information contained herein is not simply knowledge for knowledge's sake, but can be used by nurses to advance the project of New Nursing, and thus to democratise both inter-occupational relations, and relations between carers and cared for.

Nor is it simply a matter of knowledge. Another necessary factor in the attainment of freedom identified by Bhaskar is the disposition to act in one's own interests. If the information in this book can stimulate discussion within nursing, it may persuade some of the possibilities and advantages of transformation. We saw in Chapter Four that there has been a useful flow of information between occupational sociology and nursing. In some part, the purpose of this book is to continue that discourse.

This requires expansion. One of its major contentions was that the relationship between nursing and medicine cannot be fully understood by looking at these occupations in isolation. Rather, it is necessary to take a wider view that takes into account their social structural position. While there are specificities unique to the position of these occupations, they are no more immune from general social forces than any other social group. However, this does not mean that doctors and nurses are mere automatons whose actions are determined by social laws. The relationship between social structures and individuals is two-way. This allows for the possibility of the transformation of structures by social actors.

Patriarchy

Given that the most significant social structure affecting the position of nursing is that of patriarchy, it follows that improvement of nursing's position will entail the continued challenge of the constraining effects of that structure upon the working lives of nurses. Not withstanding my argument that the negative power of patriarchy has been partially attenuated over time, there is still a great deal to be done, not least in altering the occupational culture within which nurses work.

This is not simply a matter of challenging sexist ideology. There are many practical projects that could be adopted to improve the lot of female nurses. Given the number of women that are employed by the National Health Service, it is amazing how little is currently being done to accommodate them. In both the Metropolitan and Suburban Hospitals, there were no crèche facilities, no guarantees of returning to the same grade (or even getting a job) after taking time out for child-rearing, virtually no job-sharing, and little opportunity for part-time work except in areas such as night duty which tended to entail a stagnation of occupational mobility. These conditions of employment are far from exceptional.

Until women can have career structures which do not handicap them because of their gender, nursing will continue to waste experienced members, and to be characterised by an imbalance in favour of young, unmarried women. While this remains the case, it will be difficult for nursing to gain the reserves of knowledge and experience needed to compete successfully with the prodigious resources of medicine.

It is incumbent upon nurse managers to recognise the implications of the demographic makeup of the occupation, and to use their powers to promote working practices which will allow female nurses to contribute fully to the occupation.

Racism

The empirical findings about racism were, for me, the most uncomfortable in this book, in that they showed that some nurses were prepared to reproduce oppressive social structures for their own ends. Recognition of this fact tarnished the somewhat angelic image of nurses that I may have indulged in elsewhere. It reminds us once again that nurses are far from immune from the pressures of the social structures within which they are located.

While in this case, racism was used to enhance the occupational position of some nurses in relations to doctors, this should not be taken to imply that racism is not a problem for nurses. While there are few Black or Asian nurses in Ireland, the same cannot be said for nursing in Britain. Racism within nursing is self-consuming, putting Black and Asian nurses in a triple bind, in that they are subjected to the deleterious effects of patriarchy, capitalism and racism. Nor is it simply a matter of occupational cost-benefit analysis. If nurses are serious about the promotion of egalitarian relationships between themselves, patients and other health care workers, then there is no place for racist attitudes or expressions in their workplaces.

Capitalism

The constraints imposed by patriarchy are reinforced by those of capitalism. In an economic system that values profits above all else, health care will always be seen as a cost to be minimised. One of the results of this attitude is the tendency to push nursing costs down to the point where those nurses still in employment are too few and too lacking in skills to carry out the standard of care that they believe their patients deserve. This is not to say that a different economic structure could break free of the finite resources for health promotion and care available to even the richest of societies. One does not have to be utopian to assert the possibility of structuring a society's political economy in such a way that people are valued over profits.

Many nurses have been in the forefront of defending socialised health care in the face of the neo-liberal assaults that it has been subjected to over recent decades. Indeed, nurses are in a unique position in this struggle in that they are not perceived as simply grinding their own axe. Rather, their genuine commitment to the betterment of health for all is largely accepted. However, not all nurses have been persuaded of the importance of this structural issue. Nor is it hard to see why, in that, because they spend their time interacting with patients on a one-to-one basis, there is a tendency to view nursing in micro-social terms (Cooke 1993). Once again, we return to the central tenet of critical realism - that the nature of our everyday lives cannot be fully appreciated unless we take into account the social structures that enable and constrain our actions. Day-to-day issues such as skill-mixes and staffing levels are reflections of more general problems within the political economy. It is therefore only through working to transform economic structures that these issues can be resolved.

Bibliography

Abbott, P. and Wallace, C. (1990) 'The sociology of the caring professions: an introduction'. In Abbott, P. and Wallace, C. (eds) *The Sociology of the Caring Professions*. London: Falmer: 1-9.

Abdellah, F.G. and Levine, E. (1979) *Better Patient Care Through Nursing Research, 2nd Edition*. New York: Macmillan.

Aldrich, H. (1992) 'Incommensurable paradigms? Vital signs from three perspectives. In Reed, R. and Hughes, M. (eds) *Rethinking Organization: New Directions in Organization Theory and Analysis*. London: Sage 17-45.

Aldridge, J. (1993) 'The textual disembodiment of knowledge in research account writing', *Sociology*, 27(1): 53-66.

Allsop, J. (1984) *Health Policy and the National Health Service*. London: Longman.

Amos, V. and Parmar, P. (1984) 'Challenging imperial feminism', *Feminist Review*, 17: 3-20.

Anonymous (1983) 'Nursing process criticised', *British Medical Journal*, 287: 439-441.

Atkinson, J. (1986) *Changing Work Patterns: How Companies Achieve Flexibility to Meet New Needs*. London: National Economic Development Office.

Atkinson, P. (1990) *The Ethnographic Imagination: Textual Construction of Reality*. London: Routledge.

Baly, M.E. (1980) *Nursing and Social Change, 2nd Edition*. London: Heinemann.

Banton, M. (1983) *Racial and Ethnic Competition*. Cambridge: Cambridge University Press.

Barrett, M. and Roberts, H. (1978) 'Doctors and their patients: the social control of women in general practice'. In Smart, C. and Smart, B. (eds) *Women, Sexuality and Social Control*. London: Routledge and Kegan Paul: 41-52.

Bauman, Z. (1987) *Legislators and Interpreters: On Modernity, Post-Modernity and Intellectuals*. Cambridge: Polity.

Becker, H. (1967) 'Whose side are we on?', *Social Problems*, 14: 239-247.

Becker, H. (1971) *Sociological Work: Method and Substance*. London: Allen Lane.

190

Benokraitis, N. and Faigin, J. (1986) *Modern Sexism: Blatant, Subtle and Covert Discrimination*. Englewood Cliffs, N.J.: Prentice-Hall.

Berger, P.L. and Luckmann, T. (1971) *The Social Construction of Reality*. Harmondsworth: Penguin.

Berlant, J.L. (1975) *Profession and Monopoly*. Berkeley, Cal.: University of California Press.

Bhaskar, R. (1978) *A Realist Theory of Science*. Brighton: Harvester Wheatsheaf.

Bhaskar, R. (1983) 'Beef, structure and place: notes from a critical naturalist perspective', *Journal for the Theory of Social Behaviour*, 13(1): 81-95.

Bhaskar, R. (1989a) *Reclaiming Reality: A Critical Introduction to Contemporary Philosophy*. London: Verso.

Bhaskar, R. (1989b) *The Possibility of Naturalism: A Philisophical Critique of the Contemporary Human Sciences, 2nd Edition*. Hemel Hempstead: Harvester Wheatsheaf.

Bhaskar, R. (1991) *Philosophy and the Idea of Freedom*. Oxford: Blackwell.

Bhaskar, R. (1993) *Dialectic: The Pulse of Freedom*. London: Verso

Black, G. (1992) *Work in Progress: An Overview*. London: King's Fund Centre.

Blackburn, P., Coombs, R. and Green, K. (1985) *Technology, Economic Growth, and the Labour Process*. London: Macmillan.

Bourdieu, P. (1977) *Outline of a Theory of Practice*. Cambridge: Cambridge University Press.

Bourdieu, P. (1990) *The Logic of Practice*. Cambridge: Polity.

Bowman, M.P. (1983) 'Nursing by lamplight', *The Health Services*, 46: 10-11.

Boylan, A. (1982) 'The nursing process and the role of the registered nurse', *Nursing Mirror*, 25 August: 1387-1389.

Brewer, J.D. (1993) 'Sensitivity as a problem in field research: a study of routine policing in Northern Ireland'. In Renzetti, C.M. and Lee, M. (eds) *Researching Sensitive Topics*. Newbury Park, Cal.: Sage: 125-145.

Brewer, J.D. (1994) 'The ethnographic critique of ethnography: sectarianism and the RUC', *Sociology*, 28(1): 231-244.

Brindle, D. (1993) 'Doctors, nurses ... and managers', *Guardian*, 29 September: 15.

Brown, C. (1984) *Black and White in Britain*. London: Heinemann.

Bulmer, M. (1989) 'Theory and method in recent British sociology', *British Journal of Sociology: whither the empirical impulse?*, 40(3): 329-417.

Butler, J. (1992) *Patients, Policies and Politics: Before and After Working for Patients*. Buckingham: Open University Press.

Carpenter, M. (1977) 'The new managerialism and professionalism in nursing'. In Stacey, M., Reid, M., Heath, C. and Dingwall, R. (eds) *Health and the Division of Labour*, London: Croom Helm: 165-193.

Carpenter, M. (1978) 'Managerialism and the division of labour in nursing'. In Dingwall, R. and McIntosh, J. (eds) *Readings in the Sociology of Nursing*, Edinburgh: Churchill Livingstone: 87-106.

Carr-Hill, R. (1992) *Skill Mix and the Effectiveness of Nursing Care*. York: Centre for Health Economics, University of York.

Carr-Saunders, A.M. and Wilson, P.A. (1933) *The Professions*. London: Oxford University Press.

Cashmore, E. (1982) 'Black youth for whites'. In Cashmore, E. and Troyna, B. *Black Youth in Crisis*. London: Allen and Unwin: 10-14.

Chapman CM (1977) *Sociology for Nurses*. London: Balliere Tindall.

Child, J. (1986) 'New technology and the service class'. In Purcell, K., Wood, S., Watson, A. and Allen, S. (eds.), *The Changing Experience of Employment: Restructuring and Recession*, London: Macmillan: 132-155.

Clark, J. (1982) 'Nursing matters: patient advocacy', *Times Health Supplement*, 16: 9.

Clifford, C. (1985) 'Nurse-doctor relationships: Is there cause for concern?', *Nursing Practice*, 1(2): 102-108.

Clifford, J. (1986) 'Introduction: partial truths'. In Clifford, J. and Marcus, G.E. (eds) *Writing Culture: The Poetics and Politics of Ethnography*. Berkeley Cal.: University of California Press: 1-27.

Cline, S. and Spender, D. (1987) *Reflecting Men at Twice Their Natural Size: Why Women Work at Making Men Feel Good*. London: Fontana.

Code, L. (1991) *What Can She Know?*. Ithica, N.Y.: Cornell University Press.

Cogan, M.L. (1953) 'Towards a definition of profession', *Harvard Educational Review*, 23(4): 33-50.

Coleman, J.S. and Fararo, T.J. (1992) 'Introduction'. In Coleman, J.S. and Fararo, T.J. (eds) *Rational Choice Theory: Advocacy and Critique*. Newbury Park, Cal.: Sage: ix-xxii.

Collins, R. (1981) 'On the microfoundations of macrosociology'. *American Journal of Sociology*, 86: 984-1014.

Connell, R. (1987) *Gender and Power: Society, the Person and Sexual Politics*. Cambridge: Polity.

Cooke, H. (1993) 'Boundary work in the nursing curriculum: the case of sociology'. *Journal of Advanced Nursing*, 18: 338-358.

Cousins, C. (1988) 'The restructuring of welfare work: the introduction of general management and contracting out of ancillary services in the NHS'. *Work, Employment and Society*, 2: 210-228.

Cox, D. (1992) 'Crisis and opportunity in health service management'. In Loveridge, R. and Starkey, K. (eds), *Continuity and Crisis in the NHS*. Buckingham: Open University Press 23-42.

Craib, R. (1984) *Modern Social Theory: From Parsons to Habermas*. Brighton: Harvester Wheatsheaf.

Crapanzano, V. (1986) 'Hermes' dilemma: the masking of subversion in ethnographic description'. In Clifford, J. and Marcus, G.E. (eds) *Writing Culture: The Poetics and Politics of Ethnography*. Berkeley Cal.: University of California Press: 51-76.

Crompton, R. (1987) 'Gender, status and professionalism', *Sociology*, 21(3): 413-428.

Crompton, R. (1993) *Class and Stratification: An Introduction to Current Debates*. Cambridge: Polity.

192

Crompton, R. and Gubbay, J. (1977) *Economy and Class Structure*. London: Macmillan.

Crompton, R. and Jones, G. (1984) *White Collar Proletariat: Deskilling and Gender in Clerical Work*. London: Macmillan.

Crompton, R. and Sanderson, K. (1990) *Gendered Jobs and Social Change*. London: Unwin Hyman.

de la Cuesta, C. (1983) 'The nursing process: from development to implementation', *Journal of Advanced Nursing*, 8: 365-371.

Currie, C.T. (1984) 'The nursing process: revolutionary philosophy or passing phase?', *British Medical Journal*, 289: 1218-1219.

Currie, D. (1983) 'World capitalism in recession'. In Hall, S. and Jacques, M. (eds) *The Politics of Thatcherism*. London: Lawrence and Wishart: 79-105.

Darbyshire, P. (1987) 'The burden of history', *Nursing Times*, 83(4): 32-34.

Davies, C. (1995) *Gender and the Professional Predicament in Nursing*. Buckingham: Open University Press.

Davis, F. and Oleson, V.L. (1963) 'Initiation into a woman's profession: identity problems in the status transition of coed to student nurse', *Sociometry*, 26: 89-101.

Davis, K. and Moore, W.E. (1945) 'Some principles of stratification', *American Sociological Review*, 10: 242-9.

Department of Health and Social Services (NI) and the Department of Education for Northern Ireland (1992) *Integration of Nursing and Midwifery Education with the University of Ulster and the Queen's University of Belfast: Report of the Working Group Commissioned by the Permanent Secretaries Department of Health and Social Services and Department of Education for Northern Ireland*. Belfast: DHSS.

Devine, B.A. (1978) 'Nurse-physician interaction: status and social structure within two hospital wards', *Journal of Advanced Nursing*, 3: 287-295.

Dingwall, R. (1977) *The Social Organisation of Health Visitor Training*. London: Croom Helm.

Dingwall, R. and McIntosh, J. (eds) (1978) *Readings in the Sociology of Nursing*. Edinburgh: Churchill Livingstone.

Dingwall, R., Rafferty, A.M. and Webster, C. (1988) *An Introduction to the Social History of Nursing*. London: Routledge.

Douglas, J. (1972) *Observing Deviance*. New York: Random House.

Douglas, M. (1975) *Implicit Meanings: Essays in Anthropology*. London: Routledge and Kegan Paul.

Doyal, L. and Gough, I. (1991) *A Theory of Human Need*. London: Macmillan.

Du Bois, B. (1983) 'Passionate scholarship: notes on values, knowing and method in feminist social science'. In Bowles, G. and Duelli Klein, R. (eds) *Theories of Women's Studies*. London: Routledge and Kegan Paul: 105-116.

Duncan, A. and McLachan, G. (1984) *Hospital Medicine and Nursing in the 1980s: Interaction Between the Professions of Medicine and Nursing*. London: Nuffield Hospitals Provincial Trust.

Dunleavy, P. and Husbands, C.T. (1985) *British Democracy at the Crossroads*. London: Allen and Unwin.

Eagleton, T. (1991) *Ideology: an Introduction*. London: Verso.

Eastern Health and Social Services Board (1992) *Annual Report and Statistical Data*. Belfast: EHSSB.

Editorial (1981) 'Doctors and Nurses', *British Medical Journal*, 283: 683-4.

Editorial (1990) 'A suitable case for intimacy', *The Lancet*, 336: 217-18.

Ehrenreich, J. (ed) (1978) *The Cultural Crisis of Modern Medicine*. New York: Monthly Review Press.

Elias, N. (1956) 'Problems of involvement and detachment', *British Journal of Sociology*, 7: 226-241.

Elkan, R. and Robinson, J. (1991) *The Implementation of Project 2000 in a District Health Authority: The Effect on the Nursing Service*. Nottingham: Department of Nursing Studies, University of Nottingham.

Elliott, P. (1972) *The Sociology of the Professions*. London: Macmillan.

Elster, J. (1985) *Making Sense of Marx*. Cambridge: Cambridge University Press.

Elster, J. (1989) *Nuts and Bolts for the Social Sciences*. Cambridge: Cambridge University Press.

Emerton A (1992) Professionalism and the role of the UKCC, *British Journal of Nursing*, 1(1): 25-29.

Farley, L. (1978) *Sexual Shakedown*. New York: McGraw Hill.

Festinger, L. (1957) *A Theory of Cognitive Dissonance*. Stanford: Stanford University Press.

Firestone, S. (1979) *The Dialectic of Sex: The Case for Feminist Revolution*. London: The Women's Press.

Flexner, A. (1915) 'Is social work a profession?'. In *Proceedings of the National Conference of Charities and Correction*. Chicago: Hildman: 576-590.

Foucault, M. (1979) 'On governmentality', *Ideology and Consciousness*, 6: 5-22.

Freidson, E. (1970) *Profession of Medicine: A Study of the Sociology of Applied Knowledge*. New York: Dodd Mead.

Gamarnikow, E. (1978) 'Sexual division of labour: the case of nursing'. In Kuhn, A. and Wolpe, A. (eds) *Feminism and Materialism*. London: Routledge and Kegan Paul: 96-123.

Game, A. and Pringle, R. (1984) *Gender at Work*. London: Pluto.

Gaze, H. (1987) 'Men in nursing', *Nursing Times*, 83(20): 25-7.

Gellner, E. (1968) *Words and Things*. Harmondsworth: Penguin.

Gershuny, J. and Miles, I. (1983) *The New Service Economy*. London: Frances Pinter.

Giddens, A. (1976) *New Rules of Sociological Method*. London: Hutchinson.

Giddens, A. (1984) *The Constitution of Society: Outline of the Theory of Structuration*. Cambridge: Polity.

Gilligan, C. (1982) *In a Different Voice*. Cambridge, Mass.: Harvard University Press.

Glanze, W., Anderson, K. and Anderson L. (eds) (1986) *Mosby's Medical and Nursing Dictionary 2nd Edition*. St Louis: C.V. Mosby.

Goffman, E. (1968) *Asylums: Essays on the Social Situation of Mental Patients and Other Inmates.* Harmondsworth: Penguin.

Goffman, E. (1969) *The Presentation of Self in Everyday Life.* Harmondsworth: Penguin.

Goffman, E. (1983) 'The interaction order', *American Sociological Review*, 48: 1-17.

Gold, R.L. (1958) 'Roles in sociological field observations', *Social Forces*, 36: 217-223.

Gooch, J.K. (1982) 'Failure or success?', *Nursing Times*, 14 July: 1199.

Goode, W.J. (1960) 'Encroachment, charlatanism and the new professions', *American Sociological Review*, 25(6): 902-914.

Goode, W.J. (1966) '"Professions" and "non-professions"'. In Vollmer, H.M. and Mills, D.L. (eds) *Professionalization*. Englewood Cliffs, N.J.: Prentice-Hall: 34-43.

Gordon, S. (1991) 'Fear of caring: the feminist paradox', *American Journal of Nursing*, February, 44-8.

Gough, I. (1983) 'Thatcherism and the welfare state'. In Hall, S. and Jacques, M. (eds) *The Politics of Thatcherism*. London: Lawrence and Wishart: 148-168.

Gouldner, A. (1971) *The Coming Crisis of Western Sociology*. London: Heinemann.

Gramsci, A. (1971) *Selections from the Prison Notebooks*. London: Lawrence and Wishart.

Greenwood, E. (1957) 'Attributes of a profession', *Social Work*, 2(July): 45-55.

Griffiths, R. (1983) *Enquiry into NHS Management*. London: Department of Health and Social Services.

Hagell, E. (1989) 'Nursing knowledge: women's knowledge. A sociological perspective', *Journal of Advanced Nursing*, 14: 226-233.

Halson, J. (1991) 'Young women, sexual harassment and heterosexuality: violence, power relations and mixed sex schooling'. In Abbott, P. and Wallace, C. (eds) *Gender, Power and Sexuality*. London: Macmillan: 97-113.

Hammersley, M. (1990) 'What's wrong with ethnography? the myth of theoretical description', *Sociology*, 24(4): 597-616.

Hammersley, M. (1992) *What's Wrong with Ethnography?* London: Routledge.

Hammersley, M. and Atkinson, P. (1983) *Ethnography: Principles in Practice.* London: Tavistock.

Hammond, P. (1994) 'Attitude problems', *Nursing Times*, 90(9): 52.

Hannan, M.T. (1992) 'Rationality and robustness in multilevel systems'. In Coleman, J.S. and Fararo, T.J. (eds) *Rational Choice Theory: Advocacy and Critique*. Newbury Park, Cal.: Sage: 120-136.

Harré, R. (1979) *Social Being: A Theory for Social Psychology*. Oxford: Blackwell.

Harrison, S. (1988) *Managing the National Health Service: Shifting the Frontier?*. London: Chapman and Hall.

Harrison, S., Hunter, D.J. and Pollitt, C. (1990) *The Dynamics of British Health Policy*. London: Unwin Hyman.

Harvey, J. (1987) 'New technology and the gender divisions of labour'. In Lee, G. and Loveridge, R. (eds) *The Manufacture of Disadvantage*. Milton Keynes: Open University Press.

Haug, M.R. (1973) 'Deprofessionalization: an alternative hypothesis for the future'. In Halmos, P. (ed) *Professionalization and Social Change*. Keele: Sociological Review Monograph: 195-212.

Hayward, J. (ed) (1986) *Report of the Nursing Process Evaluation Working Group to the DHSS Nursing Research Liason Group*. London: King's College, University of London.

Hearn, J. (1982) 'Notes on patriarchy, professionalization and the semi-professions', *Sociology*, 16(2): 1-22.

Hechter, M. (1986) 'Rational choice theory and the study of race and ethnic relations'. In Rex, J. and Mason, D. (eds), *Theories of Race and Ethnic Relations*. Cambridge: Cambridge University Press: 264-279.

Heidegger, M. (1962) *Being and Time*. New York: Harper and Row.

Hekman, S. (1990) *Gender and Knowledge: Elements of a Postmodern Feminism*. Cambridge: Polity.

Henderson, V. (1966) *The Nature of Nursing: A Definition and its Implications for Practice, Research and Education*. New York: Macmillan.

Hirst, P. (1979) *On Law and Ideology*. London: Macmillan.

Hochschild, A. (1983) *The Managed Heart*. California: University of California Press.

Hockey, J. (1986) *Squaddies: Portrait of a Subculture*. Exeter: University of Exeter Press.

Hoekelman, R.A. (1975) 'Nurse-physician relationships', *American Journal of Nursing*, 75(7): 1150-1152.

Holton, R.J. and Turner, B.S. (1986) *Talcott Parsons on Economy and Society*. London: Routledge and Kegan Paul.

Hughes, D. (1988) 'When nurse knows best: some aspects of nurse/doctor interaction in a casualty department', *Sociology of Health and Illness*, 10(1): 1-22.

Hughes, E.C. (1945) 'Dilemmas and contradictions of status', *American Journal of Sociology*, 50: 353-359.

Hughes, E.C. (1971) *The Sociological Eye*. Chicago: Aldine-Atherton.

Hugman, R. (1991) *Power in the Caring Professions*. London: Macmillan.

Hume, D. (1969) *A Treatise on Human Nature*. Harmondsworth: Penguin.

Hunt, J. (1984) 'The development of rapport through the negotiation of gender in fieldwork among the police', *Human Organization*, 43: 283-296.

Illich, I. (1977) 'Disabling professions'. In Illich, I., Zola, I., McKnight, J., Caplan, J. and Shaiken, H. *Disabling Professions*. London: Marion Boyars: 11-39.

Illich, I. (1981) *Limits to Medicine: Medical Nemisis: The Expropriation of Health*. Harmondsworth: Penguin.

Iyer, P.W., Taptich, B.J. and Bernocchi-Losey, D. (1986) *Nursing Process and Nursing Diagnosis*. Philadelphia: W.B. Saunders.

Iveson-Iveson, J. (1981) 'Diploma in Nursing Part B Speciality (the nursing process)', *Nursing Mirror*, 2 April: 28-30.

James, N. (1992) 'Care = organisation + physical labour + emotional labour', *Sociology of Health and Illness*, 14(4): 488-509.

Jamous, H. and Peloille, B. (1970) 'Changes in the French university hospital system'. In Jackson, J.A. (ed) *Professions and Professionalization*. Cambridge: Cambridge University Press: 109-152.

Jenks, C. (1993) *Culture*. London: Routledge.

Jensen, D.M. (1959) *History and Trends of Professional Nursing*. St. Louis: C.V. Mosby.

Jessop, B. (1991) 'The welfare state in the transition from Fordism to post-Fordism'. In Jessop, B. (ed), *The Politics of Flexibility: Restructuring State and Industry in Britain, Germany and Scandanavia*. London: Elgar: 82-105.

Johnson, J. (1975) *Doing Field Research*. New York: Free Press.

Johnson, P. (1993) 'Feminism and the Enlightenment', *Radical Philosophy*, 63: 3-12.

Johnson, T.J. (1972) *Professions and Power*. London: Macmillan.

Johnson, T.J. (1977) 'The professions in the class structure'. In Scase, R. (ed) *Industrial Society: Class Cleavage and Control*, London: Allen and Unwin: 93-110.

Johnson, T.J. (1993)'Expertise and the state'. In Gane, M. ad Johnson, T. (eds) *Foucault's New Domains*. London: Routledge.

Jones, A. (1990) 'Focus on ward managers', *Senior Nurse*, 10(9): 4-5.

Jones, C. (1987) 'Handmaiden mentality', *Nursing Times*, 83(40), 59.

Kalisch, B.J. and Kalisch, P.A. (1982a) 'An analysis of the sources of physician-nurse conflict'. In Muff, J. (ed) *Socialization, Sexism, and Stereotyping: Women's Issues in Nursing*. Prospect Heights, Ill.: Waveland: 221-233.

Kalisch, P.A. and Kalisch, B.J. (1982b) 'Nurses on prime-time television', *American Journal of Nursing*, February: 264-70.

Kalisch, P.A. and Kalisch, B.J. (1982c) 'The image of the nurse in motion pictures', *American Journal of Nursing*, April: 605-11.

Kalisch, P.A. and Kalisch, B.J. (1982d) 'The image of nurses in novels', *American Journal of Nursing*, August: 1220-4.

Kant, I. (1896) *Critique of Pure Reason*. London: Macmillan.

Katz, F.E. (1969) 'Nurses'. In Etzioni, A. (ed) *The Semi-Professions and their Organization: Teachers, Nurses, Social Workers*. New York: Free Press: 54-81.

Keddy, B., Jones Gillis, M., Jacobs, P. and Rogers, M. (1986) 'The nurse-doctor relationship: an historical perspective', *Journal of Advanced Nursing*, 11: 745-753.

Kennedy, I. (1981) *The Unmasking of Medicine*. London: Allen and Unwin.

Kenney, J.W. (1991) 'Evolution of nursing science and practice'. In Deloughery, G.L. (ed) *Issues and Trends in Nursing*. St. Louis: Mosby: 67-96.

Kershaw, B. and Salvage, J. (1986) *Models for Nursing*. Chichester, Essex: John Wiley.

Knorr-Cetina, K. (1988) 'The micro-social order'. In Fielding, N.G. (ed) *Actions and Structure: Research Method and Social Theory*. London: Sage: 21-53.

Kuhn, T.S. (1970) *The Structure of Scientific Revolutions, 2nd Edition*. Chicago: University of Chicago Press.

Lash, S. and Urry, J. (1987) *The End of Organised Capital*. London: Polity.

Lewis, C.E., Resnik, B.A., Schmidt, G. and Waxman, D. (1969) 'Activities, events and outcomes in ambulatory patient care', *New England Journal of Medicine*, 280: 645-649.

Lieberman, J.K. (1970) *The Tyranny of Experts*. London: Walker.

Lipietz, A. (1987) *Miracles and Mirages: the Crisis of Global Fordism*. London: Verso.

Locke, J. (1894) *An Essay Concerning Human Understanding, Volume 1*. (Fraser, A.C. (ed)). Oxford: Clarendon.

Logan, F.J. (1976) 'The handmaiden is not dead', *The Canadian Nurse*, May: 25.

Lovell, M.C. (1982) 'Daddy's little girl: the lethal effects of paternalism in nursing'. In Muff, J. (ed) *Socialization, Sexism and Stereotyping: Women's Issues in Nursing*. Prospect Heights, Ill.: Waveland: 210-220.

McCall, G. and Simmons, J.L. (1969) *Issues in Participant Observation*. Reading, Mass.: Addison-Wesley.

McFarlane, J.K. (1983) 'Now is the time to evaluate the process', reported in *Nursing Mirror*, 28 November: 6.

Mackay, L. (1989) *Nursing a Problem*. Milton Keynes: Open University Press.

McKeown, T. (1976a) *The Modern Rise of Population*. London: Edward Arnold.

McKeown, T. (1976b) *The Role of Medicine: Dream, Mirage or Nemisis?*. London: Nuffield.

McKinlay, J.B. and Arches, J. (1985) 'Towards the proletarianization of physicians', *International Journal of Health Services*, 15(2): 161-195.

McVeigh, R. (1992) 'The specificity of Irish racism', *Race and Class*, 33(4): 331-45.

Marshall, T.H. (1963) *Sociology at the Crossroads*. London: Heinemann.

Marx, K. (1966) *Capital, Volume 3*. London: Lawrence and Wishart.

Marx, K. (1969) *Theories of Surplus Value, Volume 2*. London: Lawrence and Wishart.

Marx, K. (1970) *The German Ideology*. London: Lawrence and Wishart.

Marx, K. (1983) In Kamenka, E. (ed) *The Portable Karl Marx*. Harmondsworth: Penguin.

Mauksch, I.G. and Young, P.R. (1974) 'Nurse-physician interaction in a family medical care center', *Nursing Outlook*, 22: 113-119.

Melia, K. (1987) *Learning and Working: The Occupational Socialization of Nurses*. London: Tavistock.

Mellor, J.R. (1977) *Urban Sociology in an Urbanized Society*. London: Routledge and Kegan Paul.

Merton, R. (1968) *Social Theory and Social Structure, 3rd Edition*. New York: Free Press.

Miles, R. (1982) *Racism and Migrant Labour*. London: Routledge and Kegan Paul.

Miliband, R. (1973) *The State in Capitalist Society: The Analysis of the Western System of Power*. London: Quartet.

Milkman, R. (1983) 'Female factory labour and industrial structure: control and conflict over "women's place" in auto and electrical manufacturing', *Politics and Society*, 12: 159-203.

Millerson, G.L. (1964) *The Qualifying Association*. London: Routledge and Kegan Paul.

Millett, K. (1971) *Sexual Politics*. London: Sphere.

Mills, C.W. (1970) *The Sociological Imagination*. Harmondsworth: Penguin.

Mitchell, J.R.A., (1984), 'Is nursing any business of doctors? A simple guide to the "nursing process"', *British Medical Journal*, 288: 216-219.

Moore, J. (1988) *Letter to Audrey Emerton, Chairperson, UKCC.* 20\5\88

Mouzelis, N. (1991) *Back to Sociological Theory: The Construction of Social Orders*. London: Macmillan.

Mouzelis, N. (1993) 'The poverty of sociological theory', *Sociology* 24(4): 675-695.

Muff, J. (1982) 'Handmaiden, battle-ax, whore: an exploration into the fantasies, myths, and stereotypes about nurses'. In Muff, J. (ed) *Socialization, Sexism and Stereotyping: Women's Issues in Nursing*, Prospect Heights, Ill.: Waveland: 113-156.

Mullholland, J. and Griffiths, M. (1991) 'Primary nursing: the Ulster experience', *Nursing Times*, 87(30): 63.

Murdoch, I. (1989) 'A believer in the triumph of good', *The Independent*, 29 April: 23.

Murgatroyd, L. (1982) 'Gender and occupational stratification', *Sociological Review*, 30: 574-602.

Murphy, C. and Hunter, H. (1984) *Ethical Problems in the Nurse-Patient Relationship*. Boston, Mass.: Allwin and Bacon.

Murray, R. (1989a) 'Fordism and post-Fordism'. In Hall, S. and Jacques, M. (eds) *New Times: The Changing Face of Politics in the 1990s*. London: Lawrence and Wishart: 38-53.

Murray, R. (1989b) 'Benetton Britain' In Hall, S. and Jacques, M. (eds) *New Times: The Changing Face of Politics in the 1990s*. London: Lawrence and Wishart: 54-64.

National Board for Nursing, Midwifery and Health Visiting for Northern Ireland (1989) *The Provision of Education: A Strategy for Northern Ireland*. Belfast: National Board.

Navarro, V. (1978) *Class Struggle, the State and Medicine: An Historical and Contemporary Analysis of the Medical Sector in Great Britain*. London: Martin Robinson.

Nettleton, S. (1995) *The Sociology of Health and Illness*. Cambridge: Polity.

Northern Ireland Health and Personal Social Services (1992) *A Charter for Patients and Clients*. Belfast: HMSO.

O'Connor, J. (1976) *The Fiscal Crisis of the State*. New York: St. Martin's Press.

Oleson, V. and Whittaker, E. (1968) *The Silent Dialogue: The Social Psychology of Professional Socialization*. San Fransisco: Jossey Bass.

Oliver, D. and Walford, D., Chairpersons of the Working Party on Women Doctors and their Careers (1991) *Women Doctors and their Careers*. London: Department of Health.

Oppenheimer, M. (1973) 'The proletarianization of the professions'. In Halmos, P. (ed) *Professionalization and Social Change*. Keele: Sociological Review Monograph: 213-228.

Orem, D.E. (1985) *Nursing: Concepts and Practice*. New York: McGraw Hill.

Owens, P. and Glennerster, H. (1990) *Nursing in Conflict*. London: Macmillan.

Parkin, F. (1979) *Marxism and Class theory: A Bourgeois Critique*. London: Tavistock.

Parkin, F. (1982) *Max Weber*. Chichester: Ellis Horwood and London: Tavistock.

Parmar, P. (1982) 'Gender, race and class: Asian women in resistance'. In Centre for Contemporary Cultural Studies *The Empire Strikes Back: Race and Racism in 70's Britain*. London: Hutchinson: 236-275.

Parry, N. and Parry, J. (1976) *The Rise of the Medical Profession*. London: Croom Helm.

Parry, N. and Parry, J. (1977) 'Social closure and collective social mobility'. In Scase, R. (ed) *Industrial Society: Class, Cleavage and Control*. London: Allen and Unwin: 111-121.

Parsons, T. (1939) 'The professions and social structure', *Social Forces*, 17: 457-467.

Parsons, T. (1951) *The Social System*. New York: Free Press.

Parsons, T. (1964) 'Evolutionary universals', *American Sociological Review*, 29(4): 339-357.

Pearson, A. (ed) (1988) *Primary Nursing: Nursing in Burford and Oxford Nursing Development Units*. Beckenham: Croom Helm.

Perry, A. and Jolley, M. (1991) *Nursing: A Knowledge Base for Practice*. London: Edward Arnold.

Phillips, A. and Taylor, B. (1980) 'Sex and Skill: notes towards a feminist economics', *Feminist Review*, 6: 79-88.

Phizacklea, A. (1988) 'Gender, racism and occupational segregation'. In Walby, S. (ed) *Gender Segregation at Work*. Milton Keynes: Open University Press: 43-54.

Porter, S. (1988) 'Siding with the system', *Nursing Times*, 84(41): 30-31.

Porter, S. (1991) 'A participant observation study of power relations between nurses and doctors in a general hospital', *Journal of Advanced Nursing*, 16: 728-735.

Porter, S. (1992a) 'The poverty of professionalization: a critical analysis of strategies for the occupational advancement of nursing' *Journal of Advanced Nursing*, 17: 720-726.

Porter, S. (1992b) 'Women in a women's job: the gendered experience of nurses', *Sociology of Health and Illness*, 14(4): 510-527.

Porter, S. (1993a) 'Critical realist ethnography: the case of racism and professionalism in a medical setting', *Sociology*, 27(4): 591-609.

Porter, S. (1993b) 'The changing influence of occupational sociology', *British Journal of Nursing*, 2(22): 1113-1119.

Porter, S. (1995) 'Men researching women working', *Nursing Outlook*, forthcoming.

Ranade, W. (1994) *A Future for the NHS? Health Care in the 1990s*. London: Longman.

Rees, T. (1992) *Skill Shortages, Women and the New Information Technologies*. Brussels: Commission of the European Communities.

Reeves, F. (1983) *British Racial Discourse*. Cambridge: Cambridge University Press.

Rex, J. (1970) *Race Relations and Sociological Theory*. London: Weidenfeld and Nicholson.

Rex, J. (1986) *Race and Ethnicity*. Milton Keynes: Open University Press.

Ride, T. (1983) 'Do we understand the process?', *Nursing Mirror*, 17 August: 12-13.

Riehl, J.P. and Roy, C. (1980) *Conceptual Models for Nursing Practice, 2nd Edition*. Norwalk, Ct.: Appleton-Century-Crofts.

Robinson, J. (1991) 'Working with doctors: educational conditioning', *Nursing Times*, 87(10): 28-31.

Robinson, J., Gray, A. and Elkan, R. (eds) (1992) *Policy Issues in Nursing*. Buckingham: Open University Press.

Roth, J. (1974) 'Professionalism: the sociologists decoy', *Sociology of Work and Occupation*, 1(1): 6-23.

Rowden, R. (1984) 'Doctors can work with the nursing process: A reply to Professor Mitchell', *British Medical Journal*, 288: 219-221.

Royal College of Nursing Committee on Standards of Nursing Care (1981) *Towards Standards*. London: Royal College of Nursing.

Rueschemeyer, D. (1964) 'Doctors and lawyers: a comment on the theory of the professions', *Canadian Review of Sociology*, 1: 17-30.

Rustin, M. (1989) 'The politics of post-Fordism: or, the trouble with "New Times"', *New Left Review*, 175: 54-77.

Ryan, D. (1989) *Project 1999: The Support Hierarchy as the Management Contribution to Project 2000*. Edinburgh: Department of Nursing Studies, University of Edinburgh.

Ryan, S. and Porter, S. (1993) 'Men in nursing: a cautionary comparative critique', *Nursing Outlook*, 41(6): 462-467.

Salmon, B. (1966) *Report of the Committee on Senior Nursing Staff Structure*. London: HMSO.

Salvage, J. (1985) *The Politics of Nursing*. London: Heinemann.

Salvage, J. (1988) 'Professionalization - or a struggle for survival? A consideration of current proposals for the reform of nursing in the United Kingdom', *Journal of Advanced Nursing*, 13: 515-519.

Salvage, J. (1990) 'The theory and practice of the 'New Nursing', *Nursing Times*, 86(4): 42-45.

Salvage, J., (1992), 'The New Nursing : empowering patients or empowering nurses?'. I Robinson, J., Gray, A. and Elkan, R. (eds) *Policy Issues in Nursing*, Milton Keynes: Open University Press: 9-23.

Sawyer, J. (1988) 'Patient advocacy: on behalf of the patient', *Nursing Times*, 84(41): 27-30.

Sayers, J. (1982) *Biological Politics: Feminist and Anti-Feminist Perspectives.* London: Tavistock.

Scheff, T.J. (1992) 'Rationality and Emotion: Homage to Norbert Elias'. In Coleman, J.S. and Fararo, T.J. (eds) *Rational Choice Theory: Advocacy and Critique.* Newbury Park, Cal.: Sage: 101-119.

Schermerhorn, R.A. (1970) *Comparative Ethnic Relations.* London: Random House.

Schutz, A. (1967) *Collected Papers, Volume 1.* Den Haag: Nijhoff.

Shah, N. (1989) 'It's up to you sisters: black women and radical social work'. In Langan, N. and Lee, P. (eds) *Radical Social Work Today.* London: Unwin Hyman: 112-130.

Sharma, U.M. (1990) 'Using alternative therapies: marginal medicine and central concerns'. In Abbott, P. and Payne, G. (eds) *New Directions in the Sociology of Health.* London: Falmer: 127-139.

Silverman, D. (1985) *Qualitative Methodology and Sociology.* Aldershot: Gower.

Simpson, I.H. (1979) *From Student to Nurse: A Longitudinal Study of Socialization.* Cambridge: Cambridge University Press.

Simpson, R.L. and Simpson, I.H. (1969) 'Women and bureaucracy in the semi-professions'. In Etzioni, A. (ed) *The Semi-Professions and their Organization: Teachers, Nurses, Social Workers.* New York: Free Press: 196-265.

Slevin, O. (1989) 'Project 2000: toward implementation inNorthern Ireland', *Nursing Standard*, 40(3): 16-19.

Smith, J.P. (1981) *Sociology and Nursing, 2nd edition.* Edinburgh: Churchill Livingstone.

Smith, L. (1987) 'Doctors rule, OK?', *Nursing Times*, 83(30): 49-51.

Smith, P. (1992) *The Emotional Labour of Nursing.* London: Macmillan.

Stanley, L. (1987) 'Biography as microscope or kaleidescope? The case of 'power' in Hannah Culwick's relationship with Arthur Munby', *Women's Studies International Forum*, 10(1): 19-31.

Stanley, L. (1990) 'Doing ethnography, writing ethnography: a comment on Hammersley', *Sociology*, 24(4): 617-628.

Stanley, L. and Wise, S. (1983) *Breaking Out: Feminist Conciousness and Feminist Research.* London: Routledge and Kegan Paul.

Starr, P. and Immergut, E. (1987) 'Health care and the boundaries of politics'. In Maier, C.S. (ed) *Changing Boundaries of the Political*, Cambridge: Cambridge University Press: 221-253.

Stein, L. (1978) 'The doctor-nurse game'. In Dingwall, R. and McIntosh, M. (eds) *Readings in the Sociology of Nursing.* Edinburgh, Churchill Livingstone: 108-117.

Stein, L., Watts, D.T., Howell, T. (1990) 'The doctor-nurse game revisited', *New England Journal of Medicine*, 322(8): 546-549.

Strauss, A.L. (1987) *Qualitative Analysis for Social Scientists.* Cambridge: Cambridge University Press.

Thomstad, B., Cunningham, N. and Kaplan, B.H. (1975) 'Changing the rules of the doctor-nurse game', *Nursing Outlook*, 23: 422-427.

Tierney, A. (1984) 'A response to Professor Mitchell's "simple guide to the nursing process"', *British Medical Journal*, 288: 835-837.

Turner, B.S. (1985) 'Knowledge, skill and occupational strategy: the professionalisation of paramedical groups', *Community Health Studies*, 9(1): 38-47.

United Kingdom Central Council for Nursing, Midwifery and Health Visiting (1986) *Project 2000: A New Preparation for Practice*. London: UKCC.

United Kingdon Central Council for Nursing Midwifery and Health Visiting (1987) *Project 2000: The Final Proposals*. London: UKCC.

United Kingdom Central Council for Nursing, Midwifery and Health Visiting (1992a) *The Scope of Professional Practice*. London: UKCC.

United Kingdom Central Council for Nursing, Midwifery and Health Visiting (1992b) *Code of Professional Conduct*. London: UKCC.

Van Maanen, J. (1981) 'The informant game: selected aspects of ethnographic research in police organizations', *Urban Life*, 9: 469-494.

Vollmer, H.M. and Mills, D.L. (eds) (1966) *Professionalization*. Englewood Cliffs, N.J.: Prentice Hall.

Wacquant, L. (1989) 'Towards a reflexive sociology: a workshop with Pierre Bourdieu', *Sociological Theory*, (7): 26-63.

Walby, S. (1986) *Patriarchy at Work*. Cambridge: Polity.

Walby, S., Greenwell, J., Mackay, L. and Soothill, K. (1994) *Medicine and Nursing: Professions in a Changing Health Service*. London: Sage.

Walton, I. (1986) *The Nursing Process in Perspective: A Literature Review*. London: Department of Health and Social Security.

Walton, J. and McLachan, G. (1986) *Partnership or Prejudice: Communication Between Doctors and Those in the Other Caring Professions*. London: Nuffield Provincial Hospitals Trust.

Warren, C. and Rasmussen, P. (1977) 'Sex and gender in field research', *Urban Life*, 6: 349-369.

Webb, C. (1993) 'Feminist research: definitions, methodology, methods and evaluation', *Journal of Advanced Nursing*, 18: 416-423.

Weber, M. (1968) *Economy and Society: An Outline of Interpretive Sociology*. New York: Bedminster Press.

Webster, D. (1985) 'Medical students' views of the role of the nurse', *Nursing Research*, 34(5), 313-7.

Weitzman, L.J. (1982) 'Sex-role socialization', In Muff, J. (ed) *Socialization, Sexism and Stereotyping: Women's Issues in Nursing*, Prospect Heights, Ill.: Waveland: 157-175.

Wilding, P. (1982) *Professional Power and Social Welfare*. London: Routledge and Kegan Paul.

Wilensky, H.L. (1964) 'The professionalization of everyone?', *American Journal of Sociology*, 70: 137-58.

Wilkinson, I. (1983) 'Let's stop arguing', *Nursing Mirror*, 15 June: 29.

Williams, A. (1990) *Reflections on the Making of an Ethnographic Text*. Manchester: University of Manchester.

Williams, A. (1993) 'Diversity and agreement in feminist ethnography', *Sociology*, 27(4): 575-589.

Williams, F. (1989) *Social Policy: A Critical Introduction*. Cambridge: Polity.

Wilson-Barnett, J. and Robinson, S. (1989) (eds) *Directions in Nursing Research*, London: Scutari.

Winch, P. (1958) *The Idea of a Social Science and its Relation to Philosophy*. London: Routledge and Kegan Paul.

Witz, A. (1990) 'Patriarchy and professions: the gendered politics of occupational closure', *Sociology*, 24(4): 675-690.

Witz, A. (1992) *Professions and Patriarchy*. London: Routledge.

Woolgar, S. (1988) *Knowledge and Reflexivity*. London: Sage

Working for Patients (1989). London: HMSO.

Wright, S. (1985) 'New nurses: new boundaries', *Nursing Practice*, 1(1): 32-39.

Young, A. (1994) *Law and Professional Conduct in Nursing, 2nd Edition*. London: Scutari.

Name index

Davis, K. 164
Devine, B. 43-4, 52
Dingwall, R. 20, 42, 57, 63, 64, 72, 74-5, 76-7, 99-100, 117, 165
Douglas, J. 29
Douglas, M. 51
Doyal, L. 32-3
Du Bois, B. 65
Duncan, A. 47
Dunleavy, P. 144-5
Durkheim, E. 74

Eagleton, T. 20
Ehrenreich, J. 61, 67
Elias, N. 119
Elkan, R. 52
Elliot, P. 56, 59
Elster, J. 14, 53
Emerton, A. 69

Faigin, J. 120
Farley, L. 116
Fararo, T. 138-9
Firestone, S. 101
Flexner, A. 57, 69
Foucault, M. 142
Freidson, E. 60, 61, 69, 74, 119, 131, 142

Gamarnikow, E. 76, 99, 101, 106, 119
Game, A. 98, 114-16, 120
Gaze, H. 100
Gellner, E. 63
Gershuny, J. 143
Giddens, A. 19, 74, 94, 118, 121, 139
Gilligan, C. 167
Glanze, W. 41, 68
Glennerster, H. 146
Goffman, E. 127, 133
Gold, R. 34
Gooch, J. 48
Gordon, S. 102
Gough, I. 32-3, 140
Gouldner, A. 12

Gramsci, A. 29, 34, 138
Greenwood, E. 57
Goode, W. 57, 68
Griffiths, M. 10, 74
Griffiths, R. 118, 145-6
Gubbay, J. 5, 7

Hagell, E. 4, 68
Halson, J. 116
Hammersley, M. 10, 12-20, 23, 27
Hammond, P. 114
Hannan, M. 55, 159
Harré, R. 19
Harrison, S. 145-6
Harvey, J. 144
Haug, M. 143
Hayward, J. 48
Hearn, J. 74, 99, 101
Hechter, M. 134
Heidegger, M. 14
Hekman, S. 22
Henderson, V. 67
Hirst, P. 132
Hochschild, A. 167
Hockey, J. 20
Hoekelman, R. 43-4, 50, 98
Holton, R. 132
Hughes, D. 48-9, 53, 77, 88, 124-5, 127, 129-31, 176, 181, 182, 184
Hughes, E. 31, 130-31
Hugman, R. 65
Hume, D. 34
Hunt, J. 25, 27, 34
Hunter, H. 67
Husbands, C. 144-5

Illich, I. 61-2, 67, 182
Immergut, E. 145
Iveson-Iveson, J. 45
Iyer, P. 42

James, N. 167
Jamous, H. 60, 144
Jenks, C. 161
Jensen, D. 41

Subject index

Black
7/96